Hunza and McCarrison

—ɯ—

Advice on how to live a long and healthy life

By

John Pembrey

Published by Amazon

ISBN: 9798838650405 (paperback)

Dedications

I would like to dedicate this book to Robert McCarrison, Denis Burkitt and all the nutritional pioneers past and present who have contributed to our knowledge of how nutrition can affect our health.

Many thanks to Julie my wife and children Mark, Graham, Alex and Anna for their help and support.

Table of Contents

1

Introduction to Hunza

Hunza is a small region located in a remote beautiful valley about 100 miles long and about one mile wide. It is approximately 8,000 ft above sea level with surrounding Himalayan mountains rising to over 25,000 ft. Many glaciers in the mountains feed water down to the river Hunza which runs down the centre of this fertile valley. In the 1920's, it was situated at the very top of India and surrounded in a clockwise direction by Afghanistan, Russia, China, and Tibet. The British ruled India from 1858 until it was given independence in 1947. Because of the partition of India, Hunza then became part of Pakistan. When members of the British army first entered the then Kingdom of Hunza in the 1870's, they deposed the ruler and replaced him with a more amenable person. They reported a population of about 8,000 people who were in good health and lived long lives, although their ages could not be verified as there were no written records. The people of Hunza were noted to be slim, healthy, and athletic compared to the often obese and unhealthy relatives of the British soldiers at home. At that time in Britain, illness due to heart disease, diabetes, and cancer were common but almost unknown in Hunza.

The people of Hunza were admired and respected by several British people who visited this area. Among these admirers was General Charles Bruce. General Bruce joined the Indian Army in 1888 and served with the 5th Gurkha Rifles. He was fluent in the Nepali language. He became a veteran Himalayan mountaineer and leader of the second and third British expeditions to Mount Everest in 1922 and 1924. In 1922 his team included George

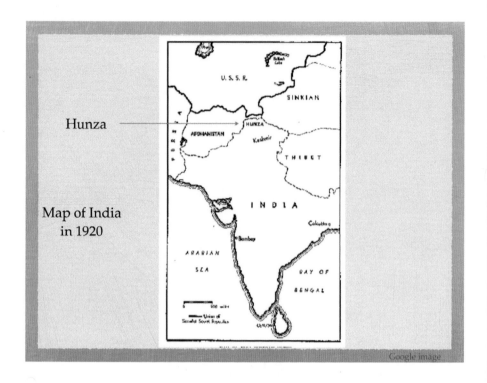

Hunza

Map of India
in 1920

Google image

Mallory. Two members of this team, George Finch, and Geoffrey Bruce, used oxygen to set a new mountaineering world record height of 27,300 ft which was only 1,700 ft below the summit of Mount Everest.

General Bruce recounted in 1928 at the Royal Geographical Society, how in 1894, he had to call up the one-time Hunza Rifles, how they left their flocks way up in the mountains, collected their kit, and went to Gilgit in one march of 65 miles of very bad country indeed. "I found the Hunza people most charming and perfectly companionable. They are as active as any people can possibly be and as slab climbers nobody in the world can beat the Hunza men. They would not prove inferior to our best Sherpa porters."

Sir Marc Aurel Stein an archaeologist who explored central Asia in four expeditions between 1900 and 1930 noted of a Hunza man: "The messenger travelled 280 miles on foot in seven days, speeding along a track mostly two to four foot wide, sometimes only supported by stakes let into the cliff wall, and twice crossing the Mintaka Pass, which is the height of Mont Blanc (15,700 ft). The messenger was quite fresh and undisturbed and did not consider that what he had done was unusual."

Other British visitors to the area remarked "Travelers and officials find these people not only fearless, good tempered and cheerful, but also possessing a marvelous agility and endurance." "Far from being nervous or morose, nearly every visitor testifies to their freedom from quarrels and exceptional cheerfulness."

It was noted that many Hunza men lived a very long and healthy life.

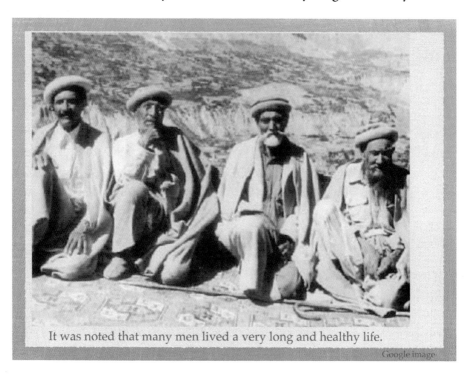

It was noted that many men lived a very long and healthy life.

Google image

2

Robert McCarrison and experiments on diet

Dr Robert McCarrison came to the Hunza area in 1904. He was born at Portadown, Ireland in 1878 and studied medicine at Queens College Belfast and Richmond Hospital Dublin before qualifying as a doctor with first class honours in 1900. He entered the Indian Medical service and sailed to India on his 23rd birthday.

McCarrison was posted as regimental medical officer to the Indian troops guarding the mountainous Northern Frontiers. He was then appointed surgeon at Gilgit which is 60 miles from Hunza from 1904 until 1911. He married Helen Johnson in 1906 and remained happily married with her until the end of his life. They had no surviving children.

While at Gilgit McCarrison did important research on sandfly fever and thyroid goitre which led to him being transferred to a research institute at Kasauli with well-equipped laboratories in 1913.

In 1912, Sir Gowland Hopkins published his work on accessory food factors which a year later were named Vitamins. McCarrison read and was influenced by this work. For centuries it had been recognised that illness could be caused by a deficiency in the diet. Eating liver was found to cure night blindness (later proved to be due to vitamin A deficiency) and pernicious anaemia (vitamin B12 deficiency). Eating citrus fruits such as oranges and lemons cured scurvy (vitamin C deficiency). Eating cod-liver oil cured rickets (vitamin D

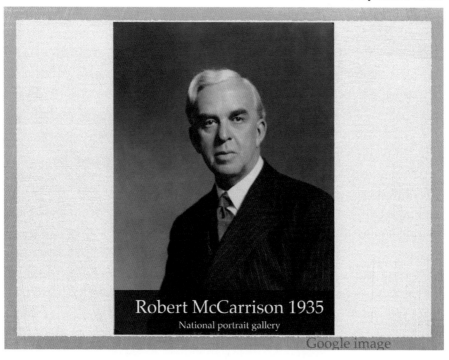

Robert McCarrison 1935
National portrait gallery

Google image

McCarrison carried out many experiments.

Effect on the growth and mortality of young rats of adding vitamins to a basal diet devoid of them but otherwise complete.

From Nutrition and Health
by Sir Robert McCarrison

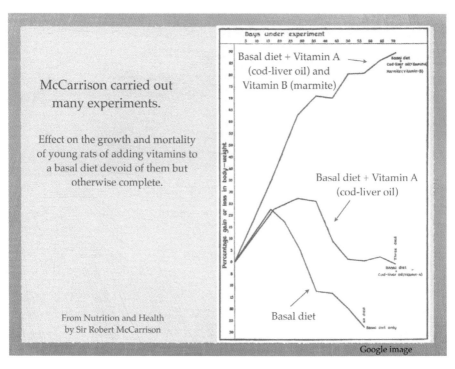

Google image

5

deficiency). Eating whole rice rather than polished rice cured Beri-Beri (vitamin B1 or thiamine deficiency) and eating yeast cured pellagra (vitamin B3 or niacin deficiency). Vitamins were not identified and named until 1913 and none were synthesised until 1935. Before this the only source of vitamins was from food. In his animal experiments McCarrison used Marmite to provide Vitamin B and butter or cod-liver oil to provide vitamin A.

During the First World War McCarrison was recalled and saw military service in the Middle East. In 1918 after convalescing from a war time illness he returned to India. He was based in a wing of the Pasteur Institute of South India at Coonoor. While there McCarrison established the National Research Laboratory of the Indian Research Fund Association (later the Indian Council of Medical Research). In 1927, he was appointed Director of Nutrition research in India and received a well-equipped laboratory and qualified assistants. He was involved in detecting deficiency diseases in the native troops and informing the government of what foods they should take to avoid these diseases. Rats were chosen to experiment with as like humans they are omnivores and like practically all human foods. Their life cycle is thirty times faster than humans so that a rat at two years old is equivalent to a human at sixty years old. They breed rapidly so that groups of rats with the same parents and therefore genes, can be studied. The rats lived in hygienic conditions with frequently changed clean straw and enjoyed daily exposures to the sun practically the whole year round.

McCarrison did many experiments comparing the effect of different diets on the growth and health of the rats. He studied the effect of feeding many rats the Hunza diet for two years which is equivalent to sixty years in humans. They all thrived and when some were killed at two years, autopsies showed no sign of illness. He compared the effect of feeding six rats on refined white flour and another six on whole wheat flour. The rats on the white flour gained very little weight and two died. The rats on the whole wheat flour thrived and none became ill or died. After ninety days, the rats on white flour had gained an average of ten grammes in weight while those on the whole wheat flour had gained an average of thirty-five grammes in weight. Adding butter (vitamin A) to the white flour in another six rats improved growth. Adding yeast (vitamin B) to the white flour in another six also produced improved growth. Adding butter and yeast to white flour produced the greatest improvement in growth and health but the results were still not nearly as good as the growth and health of the rats on whole wheat flour.

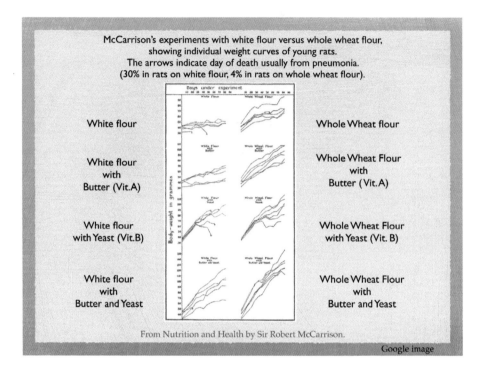

McCarrison's experiments with white flour versus whole wheat flour, showing individual weight curves of young rats.
The arrows indicate day of death usually from pneumonia.
(30% in rats on white flour, 4% in rats on whole wheat flour).

White flour

White flour
with
Butter (Vit.A)

White flour
with Yeast (Vit.B)

White flour
with
Butter and Yeast

Whole Wheat flour

Whole Wheat Flour
with
Butter (Vit.A)

Whole Wheat Flour
with Yeast (Vit. B)

Whole Wheat Flour
with
Butter and Yeast

From Nutrition and Health by Sir Robert McCarrison.

Google image

3

Research on Indian regional diets and peptic ulcer

In another experiment, seven groups of twenty rats were fed the diet of Hunza Sikh, Pathan, Bengali, Mahratta, Goorka, Kanarese and Marassi diets for a period corresponding to twelve human years. Some groups were healthier than others, but none had less disease than those on the Sikh Hunza diet. The best diet – that of the Sikh Hunzas – contained all the elements of normal nutrition. That is wholegrain bread, fresh vegetables and fruit with a small amount of milk, butter and meat. The worst diet – that of the Madrassi – was excessively rich in processed carbohydrates (polished rice), with little or no meat, milk or butter. They therefore had a diet deficient in suitable protein, minerals and vitamins.

McCarrison, when he was Director of Nutrition research in the 1920s, noted that the people in the northern Indian province of Punjab were taller and in general had better physique than those in the southern Indian province of Madras. In the Punjab, the staple diet was based on wholegrain bread and fresh vegetables with no meat but some dairy. In Madras, the staple diet was based on processed white rice and vegetables; no beef but fish and other meats were allowed. There was more air and water contamination in Madras. The incidence of certain diseases in Madras compared with the Punjab was as follows – peptic ulcer 58 times more common in Madras, worm infestation 20 times more, nephritis 10 times more, rheumatism 5 times more, cancer 4 times more, rickets 4 times more, heart disease 4 times more, diabetes 3 times more, mental illness 3 times more, anaemia 2 times more, tuberculosis 2 times more common. At the time genes and environment were thought to be the major factors in the difference between the health of these populations. However, McCarrison showed with his rat experiments that the major factor was diet.

Peptic ulcers were very common among the poor of Southern Travancore, a region at the very southern tip of India and the local doctor asked McCarrison for help. McCarrison noted that peptic ulcers were almost sixty times more common in the Southern part of India as compared with the North. He divided a healthy batch of rats into three groups. A group on the Northern Sikh Hunza diet, a group on the poorer Madrassi diet from the South and a group on the foods as prepared and cooked by the poorer people of Southern Travancore (mainly tapioca) for the equivalent of fifty human years. At the end of that time peptic ulcers were found in over a quarter of the South Travancore group (29%) and 11% in the Madrassi group. There were no peptic ulcers in a group fed on the Hunza diet. McCarrison was not sure how peptic ulcers were caused but concluded that they could be prevented by having a well-balanced nutritious diet.

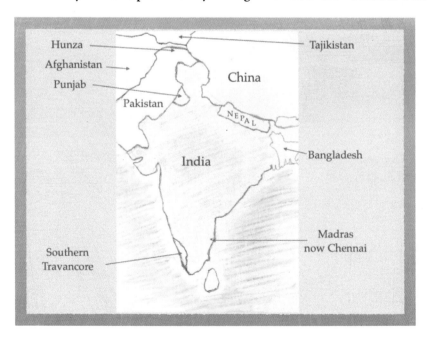

In 1922, McCarrison gave a lecture at Pittsburgh USA on 'Faulty food in relation to gastrointestinal disorder'. At that time Americans were very prone to gastrointestinal disorders especially peptic ulcers. McCarrison stated that in his seven years of association with the Hunza population he had never seen a case of dyspepsia, gastric or duodenal ulcer, appendicitis, colitis, or bowel cancer.

It has recently been found that sulforaphane, a phytochemical in cruciferous vegetables such as broccoli, cabbage, cauliflower, brussels-sprouts, kale and watercress inhibits the effect of the bacteria Helicobacter Pylori. H.Pylori is estimated to be present in over 50% of human stomachs and increases the risk of gastritis, peptic ulcer and stomach cancer. A course of antibiotics is now often given to eliminate H.Pylori in the treatment of gastritis or peptic ulcer but it looks as if a diet rich in green vegetables has a similar effect.

The Hunza diet has plenty of green vegetables containing sulforaphane, while the US diet is often deficient in vegetables but rich in processed food and animal products. The animal products produce an excess of inflammatory prostaglandins which increase acid and decrease mucous in the stomach. Cigarette smoking in the US would have aggravated the problem.

4

Comparing Hunza and English diets

In 1925 McCarrison wrote an article for 'The Practitioner' in which he stated about the people of Hunza "These people are unsurpassed by any Indian race in perfection of physique: they are long lived, vigorous in youth and age, capable of great endurance and enjoy a remarkable freedom from disease in general."

McCarrison considered the possible factors that could account for the people of Hunza's good physical and mental health into old age. Genetics, environment, and diet were all definite factors, but diet was very much under-estimated as a factor particularly in England and other rich western countries. In one of his most interesting experiments, he fed twenty rats the diet of the poor in England and twenty rats a Hunza like diet. The rats all had the same genes and environment, so that diet was the only difference.

The English diet consisted of white bread, margarine, over-sweetened tea with a little milk, boiled cabbage and boiled potato, tinned meat and tinned jam of the cheaper sorts.

The Hunza diet consisted of wholegrain flatbread (chapattis) with a pat of fresh butter, sprouted legumes, fresh raw carrots, unboiled cabbage, whole unpasteurised milk and once a week a tiny portion of meat with bone.

The rats in the English group did not thrive, their growth was stunted, they were badly proportioned, their coats were lacking gloss, they had many physical ailments. The incidence of birth defect and infant mortality was high. They were nervous and lived unhappily together. They were more likely to be aggressive and bite their carers. By the sixteenth day of the experiment, they began to kill and eat the weaker ones amongst them. They were segregated after three had been killed.

The rats in the Hunza group grew rapidly, never seemed to be ill, mated with endless enthusiasm and had healthy, birth defect free offspring. The rats were alert, happy, gentle and affectionate towards each other and their carers. The average initial body weight in both groups was 125 grams. The average final body weight after 187 days (about 6 months and equivalent to 15 human years) was 118 grams in the English group and 188 grams in the Hunza group. Six rats in the English group died of pneumonia while only one died of pneumonia in the Hunza group. After six months the rats were killed and autopsy revealed much more disease, especially of the lungs and gut in the English group.

McCarrison realised that genes and environment played a part but showed that diet was the most important factor in producing a long life with good mental as well as physical health.

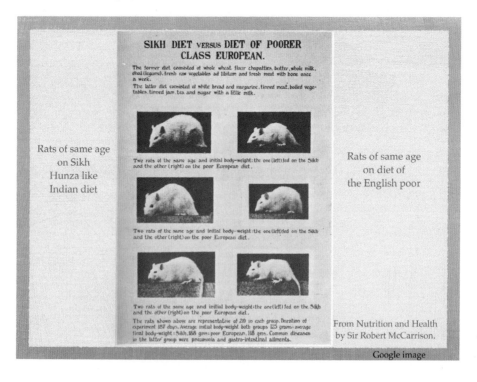

Rats of same age on Sikh Hunza like Indian diet

Rats of same age on diet of the English poor

From Nutrition and Health by Sir Robert McCarrison.

Google image

5

Hunza genes and environment

In regard to genes, the DNA of people from Hunza shows a mixture of Asian and European genes. Some people in Northern Pakistan claim to be descendants of the Greek soldiers who came to the region with Alexander the Great's army in the 4th century BC, but gene analysis only shows a small Greek component, and this may have occurred because of migration prior to Alexander the Great. There are many fine-looking people in Hunza. Hair colour can vary from black, brown, blonde, and red suggesting a mixture of Asian and European genes.

In regard to environment and lifestyle at the time of McCarrison, in the 1920's, the people were mainly poor subsistence farmers and lived in humble homes built of stone and often without windows. The houses usually had two levels with holes in the second floor and roof to serve as a smoke vent for the fire in the middle of the ground floor. The house would have been smoky and polluted during the winter but much less in the summer when fires were not necessary.

Outside the house they enjoyed beautiful scenery and fresh air. At that time, they were still living in a pre-industrial lifestyle without cars and machinery so there was very little air pollution compared with that in the industrialised West. Hunza is at a high altitude of about 8,000 ft above sea level in a valley surrounded by high Himalayan mountains. The people live in communities below terraced fields and gardens which cascade down the mountain by up to fifty levels. Below them is the Hunza river which is fed by several glaciers higher up in the mountains. As the glaciers move slowly over the underlying rocks, they produce a mineral laden silt from the crushed rock. The valley is made more fertile by a much-admired system of irrigation which includes wooden aqueducts and pipes leading away from the glaciers. Silt is carried up the side of the valley to form and replenish the soil in the terraced fields and gardens. The soil is made even more fertile by adding manure from animal and human waste. No artificial fertilisers are used. Cereal crops were rotated, and some grain was stored to be used in the winter.

The weather in winter can become very cold but there is not a great deal of snow. The temperature in the winter can be as low as minus 10 to 20 degrees centigrade. The warmest month of the year is July when the average temperature gets to around 10 degrees centigrade, but temperatures can reach as high as 14 degrees on the hottest days of summer. There is very little rainfall with an average of less than two inches in a year.

Domestic animals were mainly goats, sheep and yaks with a few cows. Grass feeding animals were favoured. Chickens were avoided as they ate a lot of the precious seeds. Wild sheep, deer, ducks, geese, pheasants and partridges were sources of meat in addition to the domestic sheep, goats and yaks. The yaks, sheep and goats could provide milk. Cows and horses were in small numbers partly because of the steep terrains but partly because they consumed more grass than sheep or goats.

Wild animals included deer such as the Ibex, wild sheep, cats such as the snow leopard and lynx, brown and black bears, wolves and foxes. Wild birds included the golden eagle, Himalayan griffon, buzzard, kestrel, crow, partridge, wagtail, skylark, thrush, finch and robin. Rodents and insects that transmit disease were rare although there were occasional cases of malaria caught from mosquitoes. The farmers got up when it became light at about 5 am and walked uphill to the fields. There were no roads or wheeled carts. All the grain and other produce was transported to the homes on the backs of men and animals such as horses or yaks. They worked physically hard until midday when they had their first meal. They had a long working day but had periods of relaxation and meditation. They went to bed when it became dark to conserve the oil required for lamps.

In summer the goats, sheep and yaks were moved to the higher mountains in search of the sparse vegetation. The herdsmen then had access to plenty of milk but those further down the valley had very little.

There was no petrol, coal, gas, or electricity. Wood, apricot kernel oil and nut casings were used as fuel. As well as fruit trees the tall and narrow Lombard poplar trees are grown as they are fast growing, provide good firewood and do not shade the vegetable gardens.

Clothing is provided by animal skins and wool but supplemented by highly prized goods brought in from neighbouring regions and countries. Imports transported with difficulty included cotton, silk, glassware, ironware including tools, knives and guns, cooking utensils, stoves and lamps.

There is an excellent community spirit and at festivals, meat was often shared out equally to each household irrespective as to who produced it. People enjoy dancing and musical events and had colourful weddings. The Hunza people speak Burushaski which is different from any other language but may derive from a mixture of the Macedonian and Persian languages. The main religion of people in Hunza used to be Buddhism but they are now mainly Shiite Muslims.

6

The Hunza Diet

In regard to diet, the people of Hunza had a mainly plant based diet with small amounts of animal products such as meat and dairy.

They had plenty of grains such as barley, millet, buckwheat, and wheat made into wholegrain chapatti bread. Wholegrain bread was eaten with each meal. Sometimes chickpeas are ground up with wheat. Sometimes beans, barley and peas are ground together.

Vegetables included potatoes (introduced by the British in 1892), beans, lentils, chickpeas, peas, carrots, turnips, squash, spinach, cabbage, cauliflower, lettuce, tomatoes, onions and garlic. They liked sprouting beans, peas and lentils. Vegetables were eaten raw or lightly cooked with water. The water in which the vegetables is cooked was drunk which provided extra vitamins, minerals and phytochemical's that are water soluble and seep out into the water on cooking.

Fruits included apples, pears, peaches, apricots, cherries, mulberries, grapes and blackberries. Apricots were eaten raw in the summer, and some were sun dried to be eaten in the winter. The kernels of the apricots were crushed to extract oil which was used in pans for cooking, lamps for lighting and stoves for heating. Oil was always in short supply and used mainly in the winter for heating and cooking meat.

During the summer, the use of fuel was avoided by eating raw vegetables and very little meat. Nuts included almonds, walnuts, hazelnuts and beechnuts.

No processed food such as refined sugar or white bread was eaten. No artificial fertilisers, herbicides or pesticides were used on the soil and plants.

Meat came from cows, yaks, goats or sheep and eaten in small amounts about once a week. Very rarely, meat came from wild animals and birds. The meat was usually boiled or cooked in butter (ghee) or apricot kernel oil and was often cooked slowly in covered pots with vegetables. Occasionally they ate sun dried meat raw.

Livestock were valuable so in the summer meat was reserved for festivals and special occasions. More was eaten in the winter when fruit and vegetables became scarce. All parts of the animal were consumed including brain, heart, lungs, liver, kidneys and gut. Bones were broken to access the marrow.

Some fresh unpasteurised milk from grass fed cows, yaks or goats was drunk. Some milk was made into butter, cheese or yogurt.

More dairy and meat was eaten during the winter as the supply of vegetables and fruit decreased. Food supplies often became low in the spring and the people and animals both became thin because of the inadequate diet.

No eggs as chickens ate the precious seeds and were banned.

Untreated water from the glaciers was drunk, herbal tea was taken without milk and no alcohol was allowed.

7

McCarrisons thoughts on diet and health

McCarrison's research and experiments led him to believe that diet rather than genes and environment, was the main factor in providing good physical and mental health. He demonstrated how many common diseases increasingly prevalent in industrial societies were caused simply by diets made defective by extensive food processing, often with the use of chemical additives. He deplored the universal consumption in Britain and America of refined white flour and the substitution of canned, preserved and artificially sweetened products for fresh natural food.

In 1926 as head of the Deficiency Disease inquiry, McCarrision submitted written and oral evidence on malnutrition to the Royal Commission on Agriculture in India. McCarrision indicated the significance of malnutrition as a cause of physical inefficiency and ill-health among the masses in India and the relationship between nutrition and agriculture. He stressed the necessity for closer co-ordination of nutritional, medical, veterinary, and agricultural research in India.

McCarrison retired from the Indian Medical service in 1935 and after thirty years in India he returned to the UK, settling at Oxford in England. After the Second World War, from 1945 to 1955, McCarrison served as director of postgraduate medical education at Oxford University.

McCarrison contributed most of his many papers and letters to the British Medical Journal (BMJ) but also published papers in the Journal of the

American Medical Association (JAMA), The Lancet and The Proceedings of the Royal Society.

In 1936 he gave a series of three lectures (Cantor Lectures) to the Royal Society of Arts in London. McCarrison noted in these lectures that in the UK, between 1920 and 1930, there were about 35,000 deaths of young people between the ages of 15 and 30 years old, mainly from infection with tuberculosis. He suspected that the high mortality was partly due to food deficient in Vitamin A. He had shown that vitamin A deficiency in rats caused structural changes in the epithelium of the mucous membranes of the respiratory tracts and lungs. Microscope slides revealed keratinisation and flaking of the epithelium and damaged cilia in the trachea. These changes would increase the risk of severe respiratory infections.

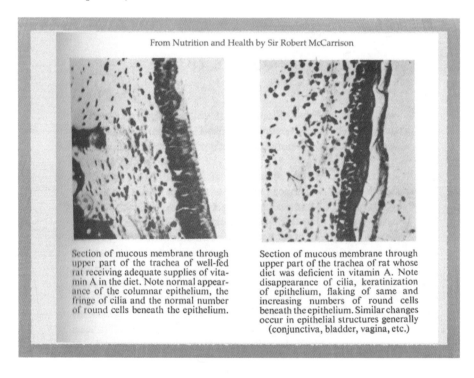

From Nutrition and Health by Sir Robert McCarrison

Section of mucous membrane through upper part of the trachea of well-fed rat receiving adequate supplies of vitamin A in the diet. Note normal appearance of the columnar epithelium, the fringe of cilia and the normal number of round cells beneath the epithelium.

Section of mucous membrane through upper part of the trachea of rat whose diet was deficient in vitamin A. Note disappearance of cilia, keratinization of epithelium, flaking of same and increasing numbers of round cells beneath the epithelium. Similar changes occur in epithelial structures generally (conjunctiva, bladder, vagina, etc.)

More young people in the cities than in the rural areas died from tuberculosis. The young people in the cities, largely because of poverty, ate less fish, liver, carrots and spinach which are the main sources of vitamin A. Other factors included lack of vitamin C from fresh vegetables and lack of sunshine because of working indoors and air pollution. This caused vitamin D deficiency. Vitamin A, C and D all give support to the immune system which helps the body fight infection. Cod liver oil and orange juice were given to children in the 1940's during the second world war because of food shortages and concern about rickets and scurvy. The cod liver oil provided vitamin A and D and the orange juice provided vitamin C. These supplements would have helped the children's immune systems fight infection and at this time there was a marked reduction of child deaths from tuberculosis.

Papworth Village Settlement near Cambridge in England was founded in 1916 by Dr (later Sir) Pendrill Varrier-Jones. It consisted of a hospital and sanatorium where patients in all stages of tuberculosis (TB) were received and treated, and a settlement where ex-patients lived with their families in a rural environment and were employed in various industries at trade union rates of pay. Initial treatment was in open air shelters. There were no antibiotics available for the treatment of TB until after 1945. When the patients' health improved at Papworth, they were moved with their family to a three-bedroom house and started a regime of graduated work. The windows in the houses were kept open to provide good ventilation and the main bedroom had a veranda where they could sit outside in the sunshine. Each house had its own garden.

McCarrison noted that in 1936 there were 400 persons in the village and that no child born there during the previous twenty years and while a member of the community had contracted tuberculosis. He put this resistance to infection down to their strong immune systems because of fresh air, sunshine and a constant supply of fresh vegetables and other good food. The assured employment of parents gave them adequate income to buy good food. During the period 1918 to 1938 records show that there were 142 families which included 368 children. None of the 108 children born in the village developed tuberculosis in any form.

The ability of a good diet to protect against infection had been noted by McCarrison during his animal experiments in India. "In the course of my own work I have seen dysentery arise in ill-fed monkeys while well-fed monkeys living in the same animal room escaped." "I have seen that the bacillus of mouse typhoid kills, on injection, over 90% of ill fed mice while it kills less than 10% of well-fed mice." In 1927 he stated "During the past two and a half years 2,463 rats, living in my laboratories under conditions of perfect hygiene, have been fed on various faulty foods, while the daily average of control or well-fed stock rats was 865. The mortality in the ill-fed animals (excluding those that were killed on conclusion of experiments) was 31%, while in the well-fed animals it was less than 1%. The chief causes of death were lung diseases, pneumonia or broncho-pneumonia and gastro-intestinal disease". "Birds are rendered susceptible to infection by anthrax when fed on food deficient in vitamin B and rats to septic broncho-pneumonia when fed on food deficient in vitamin A: guinea-pigs, when fed on food deficient in vitamin C die more readily from tuberculosis".

McCarrison concluded "The ability of the tissues to detoxify certain poisons – both bacterial and other – is reduced by diets deficient in vitamins".

8

McCarrison and Vitamin B

In 1921 Robert McCarrison published 'Studies in Deficiency Disease' He laid emphasis on the consequences of the inadequate ingestion of vitamin B in the British diet due to the extensive use of vitamin-poor white flour and the use of vitamin-poor refined sugar. He pointed out that the consumption of carbohydrate requires a greater amount of vitamin B to metabolise it which aggravates the deficiency. Later Professor J.C. Drummond confirmed that even mild deficiency of vitamin B1 gave rise to ill health especially gastrointestinal problems in many rats. Trials on American children showed that supplements of vitamin B1 produced better appetite and growth with less digestive and mental health problems.

In the 1920's and 1930's thousands of people died, and thousands were admitted to so called 'lunatic asylums' with psychosis and schizophrenic type symptoms in the Southern States of the USA due to Pellagra. Eventually pellagra was shown to be due to vitamin B3 (niacin) deficiency and fortification of white bread with B3 starting in 1938 produced a marked decline in cases and eventually a complete end of the epidemic.

In 1936 McCarrison further publicised his views in his Cantor Lectures at the Royal Society of Arts in London. I suspect these views had some influence in the decision to fortify white flour in the USA and UK with vitamin B1(thiamine) and B3 (niacin) but this did not occur until the 1940's during

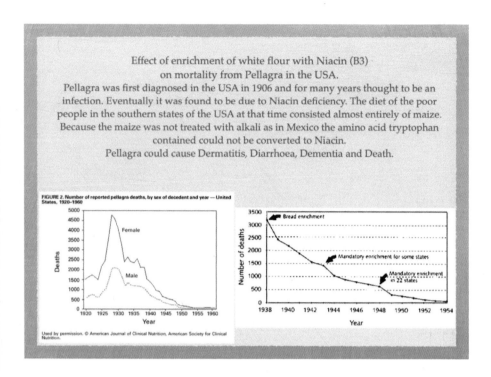

Effect of enrichment of white flour with Niacin (B3)
on mortality from Pellagra in the USA.
Pellagra was first diagnosed in the USA in 1906 and for many years thought to be an
infection. Eventually it was found to be due to Niacin deficiency. The diet of the poor
people in the southern states of the USA at that time consisted almost entirely of maize.
Because the maize was not treated with alkali as in Mexico the amino acid tryptophan
contained could not be converted to Niacin.
Pellagra could cause Dermatitis, Diarrhoea, Dementia and Death.

FIGURE 2. Number of reported pellagra deaths, by sex of decedent and year — United States, 1920–1960

Used by permission. © American Journal of Clinical Nutrition, American Society for Clinical Nutrition.

the second world war. In the USA vitamin B9 (Folic acid) was also added to white flour in 1998 which reduced the incidence of birth defects, especially spina-bifida and cardiovascular disease. In the UK it was not agreed to add folic acid until 2021.

The most common processed food is white flour made by refining wholegrain wheat. It is used to make white bread, pasta, pizza, cakes, and biscuits. The 'refining process' removes the bran outer layer and the germ centre leaving only the endosperm. The endosperm contains mainly carbohydrate which supplies energy and some protein. The removal of bran and germ take away fibre, B and E vitamins, most of the minerals and phytochemicals and the essential fatty acids including omega 3 and omega 6.

By law the white flour is supplemented with vitamins B1, B3, folic acid, iron, and calcium. Salt is also added. However, this still leaves a deficiency of many vitamins, minerals, and phytochemicals. For example, the addition of sodium and calcium to white flour while leaving a deficiency of potassium and magnesium increases the risk of hypertension. The addition of iron is

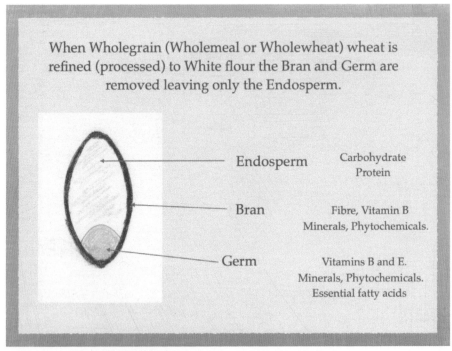

When Wholegrain (Wholemeal or Wholewheat) wheat is refined (processed) to White flour the Bran and Germ are removed leaving only the Endosperm.

Endosperm — Carbohydrate Protein

Bran — Fibre, Vitamin B Minerals, Phytochemicals.

Germ — Vitamins B and E. Minerals, Phytochemicals. Essential fatty acids

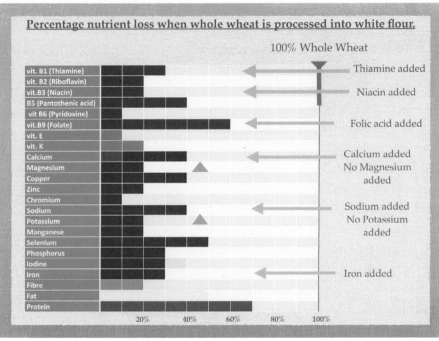

Percentage nutrient loss when whole wheat is processed into white flour.

100% Whole Wheat

vit. B1 (Thiamine)	Thiamine added
vit. B2 (Riboflavin)	
vit.B3 (Niacin)	Niacin added
B5 (Pantothenic acid)	
vit B6 (Pyridoxine)	
vit.B9 (Folate)	Folic acid added
vit. E	
vit. K	
Calcium	Calcium added
Magnesium	No Magnesium added
Copper	
Zinc	
Chromium	
Sodium	Sodium added
Potassium	No Potassium added
Manganese	
Selenium	
Phosphorus	
Iodine	
Iron	Iron added
Fibre	
Fat	
Protein	

20%   40%   60%   80%   100%

beneficial for women but may increase the risk of cardiovascular disease in men. Leaving the deficiency of iodine increases the risk of hypothyroidism and leaving the deficiency of chromium increase the risk of diabetes.

One of the factors that promoted the supplementation of white flour with vitamins and minerals was that over 50 % of the British army recruits just before the Second World War did not come up to the physical standard laid down and this was thought to be due to malnutrition in childhood. Another factor taken into consideration was that the number of people in British psychiatric hospitals had risen from a few thousand at the beginning of the 19th century to over 100,000 by 1940. By the 1940's it was known that deficiency of vitamin B1 and B3 could both cause psychosis and the symptoms of schizophrenia. In Canada, psychiatrist Dr Abram Hoffer treated over 5,000 people with schizophrenia over a 50-year period starting in the 1950's. His main treatment was to give high doses of vitamin B3 (Niacin) and vitamin C. He claimed an 85% success rate. Success meant that the patient was free of symptoms, socialising with family and friends and paying income tax (i.e. working).

9

McCarrison honoured

McCarrison received recognition for his work becoming a Major General in the Army, a Companion of the Indian Empire (C.I.E) in 1923 and a Knight in 1933. He was appointed Honourable Physician to King George V in 1935 and I suspect some of his advice has been passed on to later members of the Royal family such as the Queen mother, Prince Philip and Queen Elizabeth the second who all enjoyed a long life.

McCarrison's work was widely published in the medical press and his prizes and lectureships are witness to the honour in which he was held in England, America, and Europe. He gained the Prix Amussat of the Paris Academy of Medicine in 1914, the Stewart prize of the B.M.A. in 1918, the R.S.A. silver medal in 1925 and the Julius Wagner-Jauregg Foundation prize of Vienna in 1934.

In 1921 he made a lecture tour of the USA in which he gave the Mellon lecture in Pittsburgh, the Mary Scott Newbold lecture in Philadelphia, the Hanna lecture in Cleveland, the Mayo Foundation lecture in Rochester and the De Lamar lecture in Baltimore. He gave the Cantor lectures to the Royal Society of Arts London in 1936 and the Lloyd Roberts lecture to the Medical Society of London in 1937.

However, he was completely ignored by the British government and the medical profession in general at a time when medical thought was absorbed in the study and treatment of disease rather than on prevention and the promotion of health.

In 1927 McCarrison gave his view on the medical establishment at that time.

"Obsessed by the idea of the microbe, the protozoa, or the invisible virus as all-important excitants of disease, subservient to laboratory methods of diagnosis, and hidebound by our system of nomenclature, we often forget the most fundamental of all rules for the physician, that the right kind of food is the most important single factor in the promotion of health and the wrong kind of food is the most important single factor in the promotion of disease."

His full title when he died in 1960 at the age of 82 years was:

'Sir Robert McCarrison (1878-1960) C.I.E., M.A., M.D., D.Sc., LL.D., F.R.C.P.
Major-General I.M.S (Ret'd), Formerly Director of Research on Nutrition, India.'

In 1966 a group of doctors, dentists and veterinarians founded the McCarrison Society in honour of his work. They held meetings and published a journal called "Nutrition and Health."

10

Hunza health reviewed by doctors from USA

McCarrison had made the world aware of Hunza and in 1964 it was visited by Dr Paul Dudley White and a medical team from the USA. Dr White was an eminent cardiologist who had looked after President Eisenhower when he had a heart attack in the 1950's. He examined a group of 25 men between the ages of 90 and 110 years. Not one of them showed any sign of coronary heart disease on examination or electrocardiogram (ECG). Blood pressures and cholesterol levels were all normal. An optometrist found that all the men had healthy eyes and good vision without glasses. A dentist reported healthy teeth without decay. It was reported that in a region of 30,000 people doctors had found no evidence of vascular, respiratory or bone disease. There were no cases of cancer.

The United States National Geriatrics Society also sent Dr Jay Hoffman to investigate Hunza in the 1960's. On his return he wrote: "Down through the ages, adventurers and utopia-seeking men have fervently searched the world for the Fountain of Youth but didn't find it. However unbelievable as it may seem, a Fountain of Youth does exist high in the Himalayan Mountains. Here is a land where people do not have common diseases, such as heart ailments, cancer, arthritis, high blood pressure, diabetes, tuberculosis, hay fever, asthma, liver or gall bladder trouble, constipation, or many other ailments that plague the rest of the world. Moreover, there are no hospitals, no insane asylums, no drug stores, no saloons, no tobacco stores, no police, no jails, no crimes, no murders, and no beggars." This is a slightly exaggerated statement but does rightly suggest a remarkably low incidence of physical and mental illness. There were undoubtedly some cases of poverty and some crime. Crime was rare and punished by sending the culprit to work in the coldest, bleakest areas. Murder, which was extremely rare was punished by the death penalty.

John Clark a geologist with some medical knowledge stayed among the Hunza people for 20 months in the 1950's and reported cases of infection such as malaria, dysentery, worms, and trachoma but no mention of chronic non-infectious or non-communicable diseases such as coronary heart disease, diabetes, dementia, or cancer which were common in the West.

ll

Changing diets in the USA

While McCarrison was in Hunza during the 1920's the situation in the USA was very different. In the USA this time was called 'The Roaring Twenties'. The world was starting to recover after the First World War and the flu Pandemic which followed. The economy was recovering and wages improving. Consumer

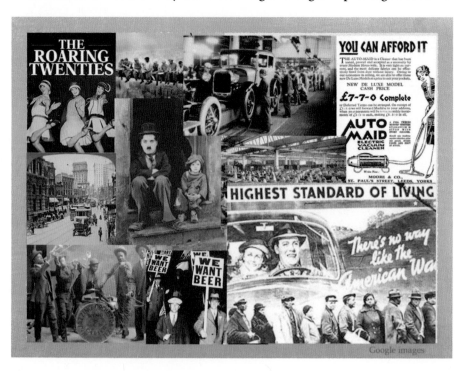

Google images

demand fuelled an increase in industrialisation with factories producing cars and labour-saving devices such as vacuum cleaners and refrigerators. People were determined to enjoy themselves after a few bleak years and this resulted in the rise of dance and jazz bands and dances such as The Charleston and Black bottom.

The 1920's in the USA marked a huge increase in advertising and a very profitable advertising industry. Partly because of advertising there was a large increase in the use of cigarettes and the consumption of meat, dairy, candy, white sliced bread, and Cola drinks. There was no advertising of alcohol as this was prohibited between 1920 and 1933.

The increase in smoking undoubtedly contributed to a rise in cardiovascular disease and cancer but the increased consumption of animal products and processed food was also a factor.

Heart attacks were uncommon in the USA before 1920 but it became the leading cause of death by 1930 when the average life expectancy in America was about 60 years. The heart attack epidemic continued with 3000 deaths

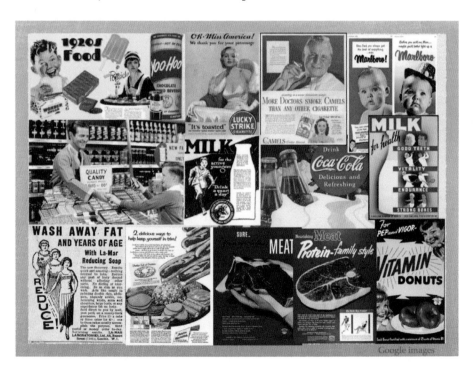

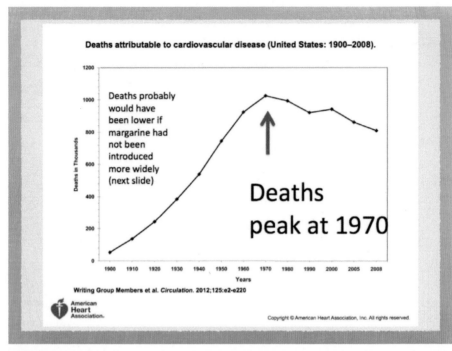

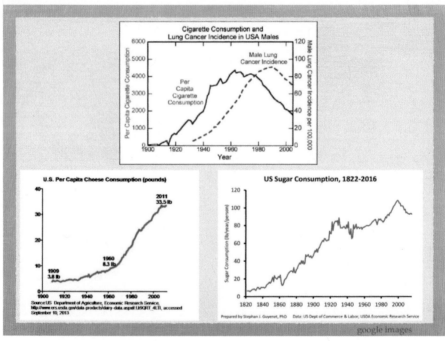

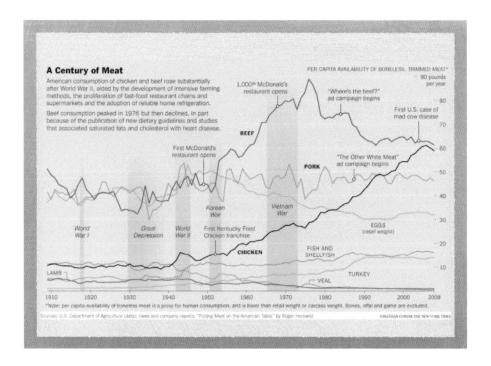

A Century of Meat

American consumption of chicken and beef rose substantially after World War II, aided by the development of intensive farming methods, the proliferation of fast-food restaurant chains and supermarkets and the adoption of reliable home refrigeration.

Beef consumption peaked in 1976 but then declined, in part because of the publication of new dietary guidelines and studies that associated saturated fats and cholesterol with heart disease.

PER CAPITA AVAILABILITY OF BONELESS, TRIMMED MEAT*

Note: per capita availability of boneless meat is a proxy for human consumption, and is lower than retail weight or carcass weight. Bones, offal and game are excluded.

Sources: U.S. Department of Agriculture (data); news and company reports; "Putting Meat on the American Table," by Roger Horowitz   JONATHAN CORUM/THE NEW YORK TIMES

from heart attacks in 1930, 500,000 deaths in 1960 and over one million deaths in 1970. The graphs above show the increase in deaths from cardiovascular disease in the early 1900's together with graphs showing the increases in cigarette smoking, cheese representing dairy, sugar, and meat during that time. Note that they are per capita so take account of any increase in population.

The graph above shows the astonishing increase in meat consumption per person in the USA during the early 1900's. The increase was due to increased wealth, advertising, increase in production of meat and the ability to transport it by lorry and train. The meat could be stored in refrigerators. The meat industry became very wealthy and powerful. To encourage the already profitable meat and dairy industries government subsidies were given.

The increase of animal products in the USA diet meant that people were having a great deal more saturated fat and cholesterol in their diets. They were also consuming more refined sugar and refined bread.

12

The cause of heart attacks

The cause of heart attacks and most strokes is atherosclerosis. This can also be called atheroma or cardiovascular disease. It is often referred to as furring up of the arteries. It starts with a stiffening of the artery due to calcification of the media layer which contains muscle and elastic tissue. The main cause of calcification of the arteries is a high dairy intake of milk, butter, and cheese. Dairy products have a high calcium content but a low magnesium content. Magnesium which is mainly in plants helps to keep calcium soluble and if there is a high calcium to magnesium ratio, calcium can be deposited in the arteries. A high consumption of the mineral phosphorus also increases the risk of arterial calcification. Phosphorus is naturally present in most foods but in much higher amounts in meat and dairy products. It is also often added as a preservative to meat, dairy products and cola drinks. The blood pressure is raised in the calcified stiffened arteries and stress at the branching of arteries can cause fissures to develop. Cholesterol is involved with healing wounds and so accumulates at the fissure and is incorporated into the inner layer as fatty streaks and then plaques.

The most common cause of angina is a narrowing of the artery so that insufficient oxygen is carried to the heart muscle. The most common cause of a heart attack is rupture of the plaque which causes thrombosis of the blood and a blocked artery. The severity of a heart attack depends on which artery is blocked. If a major artery is blocked it may cause sudden death. If smaller vessels block the person may survive. If the blockage is permanent the muscle supplied dies and weakens the heart. Modern cardiac treatment aims to try and unblock the artery before the muscle dies and insert a stent to prevent further blockage at that site.

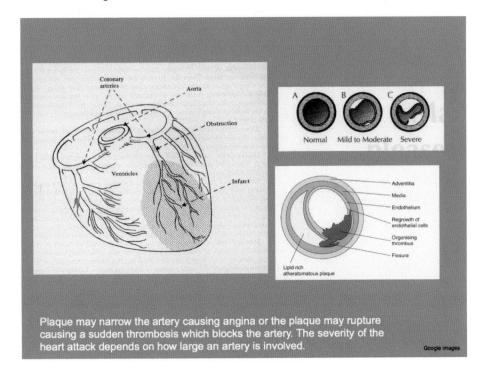

Plaque may narrow the artery causing angina or the plaque may rupture causing a sudden thrombosis which blocks the artery. The severity of the heart attack depends on how large an artery is involved.

Google images

People are more at risk of a heart attack if they consume an excess of animal products and fried or processed food. Animal products have large amounts of saturated fat and cholesterol. Fried and processed food contain trans-fats.

A high consumption of cholesterol increases the plaque size. A deficiency of essential fatty acids such as omega 3 makes the surface of the plaque fragile and more likely to rupture. The recommended daily intake of cholesterol is 200 to 300 mg a day. One egg contains 225 mg. One portion of cheddar cheese contains 70 mg, and a small 10 g pat of butter contains 26 mg. In the 1970's it was estimated that the average adult in the USA consumed about

Atherosclerosis of Arteries

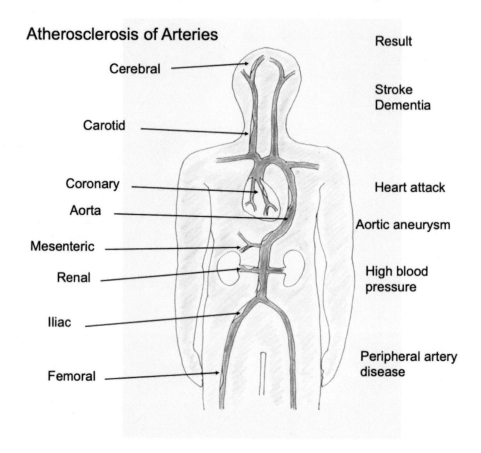

Cerebral

Carotid

Coronary

Aorta

Mesenteric

Renal

Iliac

Femoral

Result

Stroke
Dementia

Heart attack

Aortic aneurysm

High blood
pressure

Peripheral artery
disease

800 mg of cholesterol daily. 45% from eggs, 35% from meat and 20% from dairy.

Trans-fats are produced when vegetable oils are heated as in frying or are hydrogenated to make them solid as in margarine. Most processed foods contain trans-fats and they have been found to increase the risk of heart attacks even more than saturated fat as this study from Harvard School of Public Health shows.

Saturated Fat as Compared with Unsaturated Fats and sources of Carbohydrates in Relation to Risk of Coronary Heart Disease : A Prospective Cohort Study.

Published in the Journal of the American College of Cardiology 2015
Authors: Yanping Li, Phd, Adela Hruby, Phd, MPH, Adam Bernstein, MD, Scd, Sylvia Ley Phd, Dong Wang, MD, Stephanie Chiuve, Scd, Laura Sampson, RD, Kathryn Rexrode MD, MPH, Eric Rimm, Scd, Walter Willett, MD, DRPH and Frank Hu,MD, Phd.
Department of Nutrition, Harvard T.H.Chan School of Public Health, Boston,Massachusetts,USA.

This is an extremely large and important study which shows the relationship between different fats and mortality from coronary heart disease.
The researchers followed 127,536 people (84,628 women from the Nurse's Health Study 1980 to 2010 and 42,908 men from the Health Professionals Follow-up Study 1986 to 2010 who were free of diabetes, cardiovascular disease and cancer at baseline).
Diet was assessed by a questionnaire every 4 years.
During 24 to 32 years of follow up there were 7,667 cases of Coronary heart disease (4,931 nonfatal and 2,736 fatal myocardial infarcts)

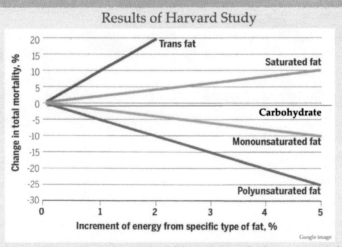

Results of Harvard Study

Relation between increasing intakes of Trans, Saturated, Monounsaturated and Polyunsaturated fats (compared isocalorically with Carbohydrate) in relation to total mortality from coronary heart disease.
Trans fats were shown to increase the risk even more than saturated fat.
Monounsaturated and polyunsaturated fats decreased the risk.

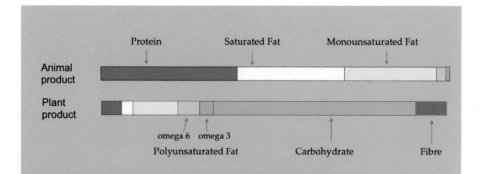

The animal products such as meat or cheese contain more saturated fat but less polyunsaturated fat. The animal products do not contain carbohydrate or fibre. Saturated fat is solid at room temperature and stable if heated. Monounsaturated fat is like a thick oil and also heat stable. Polyunsaturated fats (omega 6 and omega 3) are liquid oils and not heat stable. Omega 3 is more liquid than omega 6 and the most unstable when heated. The unstable polyunsaturated fats can be partially converted into trans-fats when heated to a high temperature as in frying or if hydrogenated to make them solidify as in margarine or shortening.

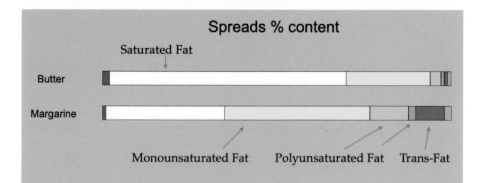

Margarine was thought to be more healthy than butter when introduced as it was made from plant fats and unlike butter did not contain cholesterol. However the polyunsaturated plant fats that margarine is made of are oily liquids in their natural state and have to be hydrogenated to make them into a spreadable solid. This hydrogenation converts most of the polyunsaturated fats into Trans-fats which we now know increase the risk of coronary heart disease even more than saturated fat.
In mediterranean countries which have a low incidence of coronary heart disease neither butter or margarine is commonly used. Natural cold pressed olive oil is often used on bread instead.
It is worth trying to avoid the consumption of butter and margarine or use very little.

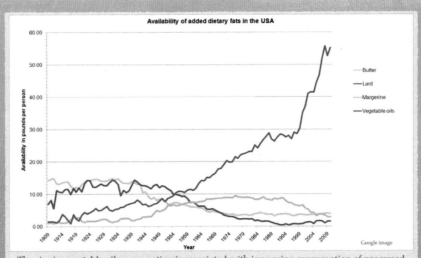

The rise in vegetable oil consumption is associated with increasing consumption of processed
and fried food at home and from fast food takeaways.

It is the main reason for the increasing intake of Trans-fats.

The main vegetable oils are from Palm, Soybean, Sunflower, Rapeseed and Olive. The production
of vegetable oils for cooking, dressings and biofuel is a major cause of deforestation.

13

The Seven Countries Study

In the 1950's research especially the Seven Countries study led by the American physiologist Ancel Keys, had suggested that diet was an important factor. A high intake of saturated fat and cholesterol in animal products was shown to increase the risk of a heart attack. The fats in plants and fish reduced the risk of a heart attack.

The study started in 1958. 12,763 healthy men with no history of heart disease between the ages of 40 and 60 years of age were studied. About 1,000 to 2,000 men in each country. Their diets were analysed. weight, blood pressure and blood cholesterol were measured, and the incidence of heart attacks noted.

After ten years of the study Crete had the lowest number of men dying from a heart attack. Only 9 men died in Crete compared with 424 in the USA. Just as many of the men smoked in Crete as the USA but saturated fat in the USA was on average about 18% of their diet compared with about 6% in Crete. The average blood cholesterol levels in the USA were about 6.2 mmol/litre while they were 5.2 in Crete. The men in Crete had more total fat than those in the USA but almost all of this was the healthy monounsaturated and polyunsaturated fat from plants which reduced cholesterol levels.

The main difference in diet was that in the USA animal products consumed accounted for 35% of their diet whereas animal products in Crete accounted for only 5%.

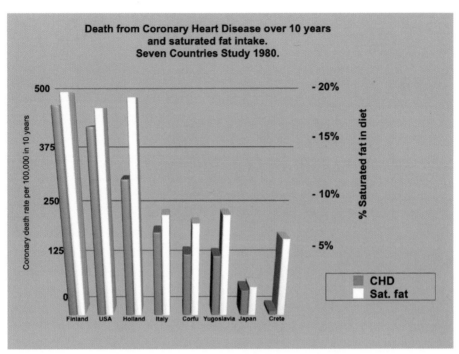

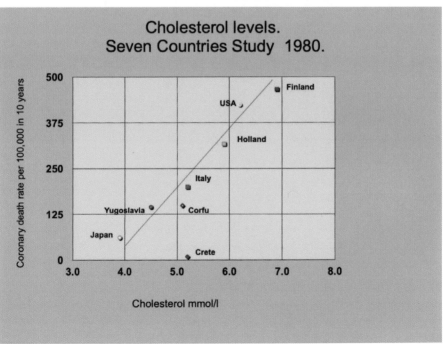

1987	Food gms/day	Crete	USA
♦	Fruit	464	233
	Bread	390	97
	Vegetables	191	171
	Pulses	30	1
	Alcohol	15	6
♦	Fat	95	33
♦	Meat	35	273
	Fish	18	3
♦	Animal based	5%	35%
	Plant based	95%	65%
Deaths from coronary heart disease per 100.000 people over 10 years in Seven Countries study 1980.		9	424

The men from Finland had the highest death rate from heart attacks. In 1991 thirty years after the start of the study 50% of the Cretan men were alive. None of the men from Finland had survived. The Mediterranean diet was advised and became very popular for a while.

14

Support from Cardiologists

Dr Christiaan Barnard, a South African cardiac surgeon, and Professor of Surgery at the University of Cape Town, performed the first human heart transplant in 1967. He recognized the importance of a plant-based diet in preventing heart disease. In his book ' 50 ways to a healthy heart' in 1990 he wrote "It's so simple. Learn to live like the people of Crete. Heart disease is practically unknown there. A comparative study found that heart problems occur 95% less often than in the United States or Europe. A test check-up done by the American Society for Prevention found that patients with heart problems who changed their diets to the Crete Method were able to reduce their heart attack risk by 70%. Astoundingly, the positive effects of the Crete Method were clearly measurable within six weeks of the dietary change."

Americans had already been advised by the American Heart Association and US Government in 1956 to reduce their consumption of beef, eggs, butter, cheese, and refined sugar. They had also been told to reduce cigarette smoking. Beef and butter consumption decreased but the consumption of leaner meat such as chicken increased, and margarine consumption increased as a substitute for butter. Margarine was made from hydrogenated vegetable oils and therefore had no cholesterol but the process of solidifying the vegetable oils by hydrogenation produced abnormal fats called trans-fats. These were found to be even more unhealthy than saturated fat and cholesterol. People stopped cooking in animal fat such as lard and butter and started using vegetable oils. Unfortunately, heating vegetable oils to high temperatures also produces trans-fats.

In the years following the seven countries study there have been many confusing and misleading trials sponsored by the food industry as it tried to defend its products. Saturated fat has been made more acceptable often by substituting saturated fat from plant products in trials. Saturated fat is in all plants and animal products. The saturated fat in plants is much less and accompanied by more of the healthy mono-unsaturated and polyunsaturated fats. In animal products there is much more saturated fat and less monounsaturated and polyunsaturated fat. Meat, dairy and eggs all contain cholesterol, and this does raise cholesterol levels in the blood especially of the more harmful low density lipoprotein cholesterol (LDL).

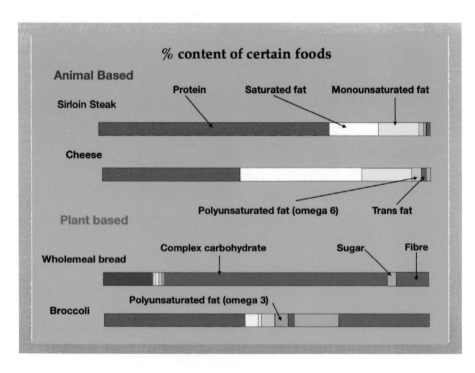

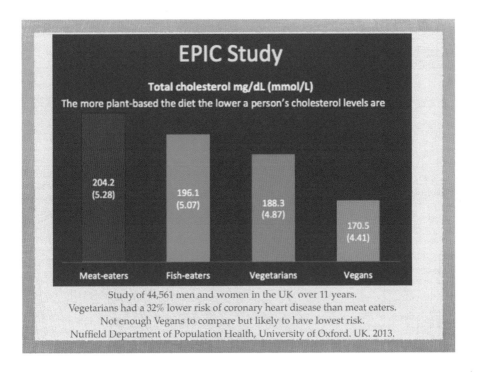

Study of 44,561 men and women in the UK over 11 years.
Vegetarians had a 32% lower risk of coronary heart disease than meat eaters.
Not enough Vegans to compare but likely to have lowest risk.
Nuffield Department of Population Health, University of Oxford. UK. 2013.

Recent trials have suggested that cholesterol in food does not make any difference to blood cholesterol levels, yet vegans are known to have lower cholesterol levels than meat and dairy consumers. It is a fact that only about 15% of the body's cholesterol is required from the diet and about 85% is synthesized by the liver. However, cholesterol consumed from the diet still makes a significant difference to blood cholesterol levels. Statins were introduced in the 1980's and are effective in reducing the amount of cholesterol produced by the liver. Unfortunately, this allows many people to continue with a poor diet because they are reassured by their low blood cholesterol levels. Some patients and doctors strive for too low a blood cholesterol level and it must be remembered that a certain amount of both saturated fat and cholesterol is required by humans. Saturated fat acts as a store of energy and subcutaneous fat insulates the body. It also stores fat soluble vitamins and hormones. Cholesterol has many useful functions including strengthening cell membranes and helping the immune system by acting as an antioxidant. It is required for making vitamin D, steroid and sex hormones. About 25% of the body cholesterol is in the brain and essential for optimal brain function. A high amount of oxidised cholesterol increases the risk of artery narrowing (atherosclerosis) which causes heart disease, strokes, and dementia but a very low cholesterol may cause depression or dementia and seems to increase the risk of diabetes. A very low blood cholesterol does reduce the risk of a heart attack but is associated with increased mortality from other causes.

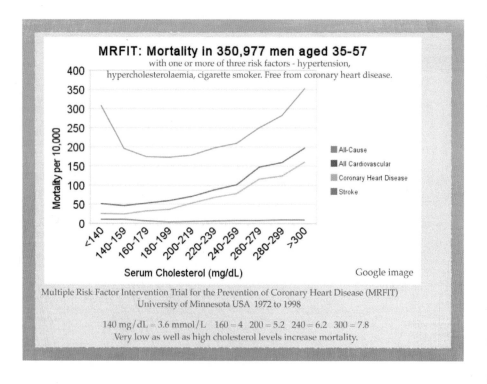

MRFIT: Mortality in 350,977 men aged 35-57
with one or more of three risk factors - hypertension, hypercholesterolaemia, cigarette smoker. Free from coronary heart disease.

Multiple Risk Factor Intervention Trial for the Prevention of Coronary Heart Disease (MRFIT)
University of Minnesota USA 1972 to 1998

140 mg/dL = 3.6 mmol/L   160 = 4   200 = 5.2   240 = 6.2   300 = 7.8
Very low as well as high cholesterol levels increase mortality.

Despite its critics I think the Seven Countries Study by Ancel Keys has a lot of merit. He perhaps could have included an excess of animal protein as a risk factor and that an excess of saturated fat and cholesterol was merely an indication that an excess of animal products increases the risk of coronary heart disease.

Cardiologists in the USA confirmed that lowering saturated fat and cholesterol in clinical practice reduced symptoms and cardiac angiograms showed an improvement of coronary arteries. Dr Dean Ornish, a cardiologist at the University of California, published his book 'Dr Dean Ornish's Program for Reversing Heart Disease' in 1990 in which he states:

"There were many research studies proving that diets high in fat and cholesterol cause blood cholesterol levels and blood pressure to go up, whereas low-fat, low-cholesterol diets cause blood cholesterol levels and blood pressure to go down. Epidemiology studies showed that high blood cholesterol levels increase the risk of heart disease in virtually all countries throughout the world," "The first coronary bypass operation was performed in the USA in 1967. By 1987 there were over 200,000 operations a year. Balloon angioplasty in the USA started in 1977 and by 1983 there were 32,000 procedures. In 1988 this had increased to 200,000 procedures." "If I perform bypass surgery on a patient, the insurance company will pay at least 30.000 dollars. If I perform a balloon angioplasty on a patient, the insurance company will pay at least 7.500 dollars. If I spend the same amount of time teaching a heart patient about nutrition and stress management techniques, the insurance company will pay no more than 150 dollars. If I spend that time teaching a well person how to stay healthy, the insurance company will not pay at all."

Dr Caldwell Esselstyn was a cardiac surgeon at the prestigious Cleveland Clinic in Ohio from 1969. He noted that a diet high in fat and cholesterol had been shown to cause coronary heart disease in animals and humans. In 1984 he gave up meat and dairy. His cholesterol dropped from 185 to 119 mg/dL. He then started advising his patients with angina and proven coronary heart disease. They were advised a plant-based diet, avoiding anything with a face or mother. As well as avoiding meat, poultry, fish, and eggs he advised avoiding all oils and refined grains. All vegetables were to be increased and supplements were given of vitamins B12 and Vitamin D, Omega-3 fatty acids and statins if required. There were many cases of dramatic improvement in his patients. Mortality from all causes reduced by 49%. In 2007 his book 'Prevent and Reverse Heart Disease' was published and became 'The New York Times Bestseller'.

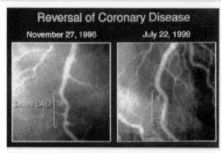

Reversal of Coronary Disease
November 27, 1996   July 22, 1999

Dr Caldwell Esselstyn a cardiologist in the USA showed that changing to a plant based diet could treat and reverse coronary disease.

Figure 1 *Coronary angiograms of the distal left anterior descending artery before (left bracket) and after (right bracket) 32 months of a plant-based diet without cholesterol-lowering medication, showing profound improvement.*

Google Image

Dr. Esselstyn study from 'Prevent and Reverse Heart Disease'.

15

The Karelia Project

The Karelia project in Finland showed the value of education and a change of diet with less saturated fat, cholesterol, and salt in reducing the mortality from heart attacks.

North Karelia is an eastern province of Finland containing about 180,000 people. In the 1970's Finnish men had the world's highest rate of coronary heart disease mortality. North Karelia's rate was 40% worse than that. About 1,000 heart attacks a year occurred, and half of these attacks were in men under 65. 40% were fatal. 1 in 10 of the men and women in North Karelia aged between 45 and 60 years were on disability leave due to heart disease.

In North Karelia in 1970 there was a high incidence of smoking – 52%. There was a high consumption of animal products and low consumption of fruit and vegetables. Full cream milk was drunk, and local butter and cream were popular. There was a high consumption of sausages, pork, and fatty meats. Salt intake was high. The citizens of North Karelia petitioned the Finnish Government in 1971 and a project was sponsored by the Government and the World Health Organization. The project was directed by Dr Pekka Puska a 27-year-old with a master's degree in social science. He arranged talks at schools and community centers. Advice was given in pamphlets, newspaper articles, radio, and TV. Groups of housewives educated members. Recipes were changed at home, schools, and cafes. Free healthy school meals were given. Food manufacturers lowered the fat and salt in sausages, bread etc. Subsidies were given to dairy farmers who switched to growing berries and rapeseed. Exercise was encouraged and more sporting facilities provided. For example, bike paths and cross-country ski parks were developed. They introduced Pansalt, a salt substitute which has 40% less sodium than normal salt. The sodium was replaced by 28% potassium and 12% magnesium. Pansalt was put in their processed foods and replaced table salt.

The Karelia project ran for 25 years from 1972 to 1997 and was a great success.

The average blood pressure dropped from 150/90 to 140/85.

The average blood cholesterol level dropped from 6.9 to 5.7.

The heart attack rate in males 35 to 64 years reduced by 70%

Heart attack deaths reduced by 73%

Lung cancer deaths reduced by 71%.

All cancer deaths reduced by 44%.

The rest of Finland joined the project in 1977.

From 1971 to 1979 the project cost $1.75 million.

The reduced number of heart attacks and strokes saved $2 million.

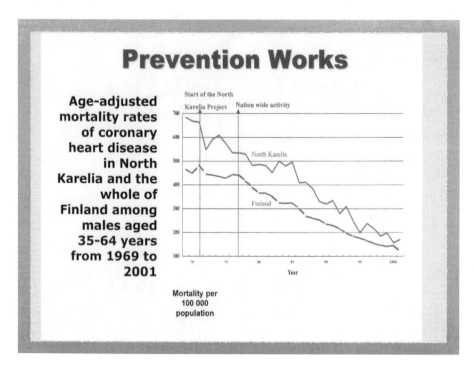

Prevention Works

Age-adjusted mortality rates of coronary heart disease in North Karelia and the whole of Finland among males aged 35-64 years from 1969 to 2001

Mortality per 100 000 population

Reduction in disability pensions saved $4 million.

Most importantly.

There was a huge reduction in human suffering and loss because people were healthier.

16

USA advertising and excess protein

Because of the intense lobbying and advertising by the meat, egg, and dairy industries and because they were very profitable the American government were not as critical as the medical advice warranted and they even encouraged animal product consumption by giving large subsidies on animal feed, milk and butter but not on vegetables and fruit.

One of the problems was that the advertisers could claim that certain parts of animal products were nutritious. Meat is correctly advertised as having good quality protein containing all the essential amino acids, but they never mention the saturated fat, cholesterol, hormones, and the side effects of excess protein. Dairy products, milk, butter, and cheese are correctly advertised as having plenty of calcium but there is no mention of the growth and sex hormones and very low magnesium content. The high calcium and low magnesium ratio increase the risk of arterial calcification, hypertension and cardiovascular disease and the hormones increase the risk of cancer.

A high intake of Methionine, an amino acid which is much higher in animal protein can upset methylation and increase the risk of mental health problems, birth defects, miscarriages, cardiovascular disease and cancer. (See Chapter 20 (a) for more details.)

Animal protein produces a lot more inflammatory prostaglandins than plant protein which increase the risk of many western illnesses. (See Chapter 20 (c))

Animal protein has far less phytochemicals and antioxidants than plant protein and no fibre, so there is less support for the immune system.

People should note that the large boned and well-muscled cows and yaks get all the protein and calcium they need from plants in the form of grass. There are many examples of successful boxers, wrestlers and body builders who are vegan. For example, David Haye past cruiser weight boxing world champion and Barry du Plessis bodybuilder and Mr. Universe 2014. Successful athletes who are vegan and so get all their protein from plants include Wimbledon tennis champions Venus Williams and Novak Djokovic, football star Lionel Messi and motor racing world champion Lewis Hamilton.

Unfortunately, people in the USA are still being persuaded that they must have more protein and that this protein is best provided by animals. Young athletes are encouraged to have whey powder and protein bars and the elderly are often given animal-based protein supplements.

A certain amount of protein is required daily. Plants do not contain as much protein as animal products, and it is not as complete in essential amino acids. However, there are many combinations of vegetables which provide all the essential amino acids, and it is possible to get all the protein you need from a purely plant based (vegan) diet. It is estimated that the average adult human requires about 50 grams of protein a day.

The people in Hunza had adequate protein (about 50g) but in the 1920's only 1% was from animal products, 99% was for plant foods.

In the USA people tended to have much more than 50g of protein daily and sometimes double that amount. It was also mainly from animal products.

Any excess of protein cannot be stored so it is converted to acid metabolites such as sulphuric acid, urea, and uric acid. This causes a metabolic acidosis which the body corrects by taking calcium and phosphate from the bones and excreting them together with the acid protein

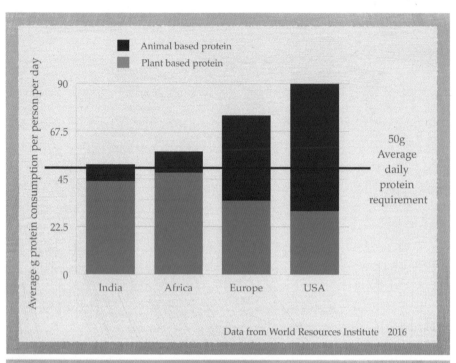

Data from World Resources Institute   2016

Protein in Food

Animal	Protein per 100g	Plant	Protein per 100g
Whey powder	97 g	Peanuts	26 g
Chicken	31 g	Almonds	21 g
Beef	26 g	Peas	5 g
Cheese	25 g	Beans	5 g
Salmon	20 g	Cabbage	1 g
Cod	18 g		
Egg white	11 g		

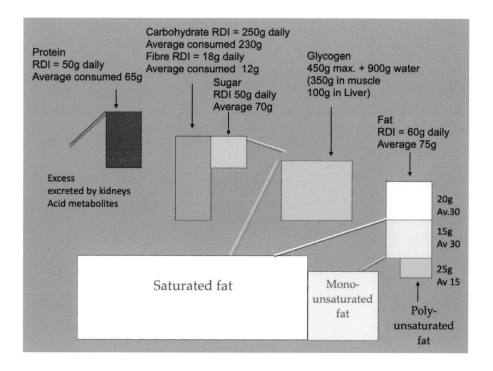

Protein
RDI = 50g daily
Average consumed 65g

Carbohydrate RDI = 250g daily
Average consumed 230g
Fibre RDI = 18g daily
Average consumed 12g
Sugar
RDI 50g daily
Average 70g

Glycogen
450g max. + 900g water
(350g in muscle
100g in Liver)

Fat
RDI = 60g daily
Average 75g

Excess
excreted by kidneys
Acid metabolites

20g
Av.30

15g
Av 30

25g
Av 15

Saturated fat

Mono-
unsaturated
fat

Poly-
unsaturated
fat

metabolites in the urine. This increases the risk of kidney stones, gout and osteoporosis.

The body can store the sugar in carbohydrate as glycogen in the liver and muscles. If the glycogen stores are full, then it is converted to fat.

Saturated fat and monounsaturated fat can also be stored but not polyunsaturated fat which includes Omega 6 and Omega 3.

17

Food can be a poison: causes of Western illnesses

The people in Hunza also have meat and milk but in much smaller amounts.

"Poison is in everything, and nothing is without poison. The dosage makes it either a poison or a remedy" This is a quote by Paracelsus a 16th century Swiss physician.

Oxygen is essential to life and a remedy when supplied at 20% in air. However, 100% oxygen for other than a short period is a poison and harms the body. Water is essential to life and a remedy for dehydration, but an excess of water can act as a poison. It is a well-known fact that water intoxication kills more people running marathons than dehydration. The same principle applies to the food we eat. An excess of protein, fat, sugar, and hormones can all act as a poison.

The American public should have been strongly advised for the sake of their health to simply reduce all animal-based products and increase plant-based products, stop smoking, and have whole foods rather than processed food. The message is getting through to some people but there are still many who have poor health because they do not take this advice.

The high animal diet in the USA causes an excessive consumption of protein, saturated fat, cholesterol, sex and growth hormones and inflammatory prostaglandins. Because of the reduced consumption of vegetables there is a risk of deficiency in fibre, vitamins especially vitamin C and folic acid, minerals, and phytochemicals. There are far less antioxidants and phytochemicals in animal-based foods compared with plant-based foods.

The high amount of processed food in the USA diet causes an excessive consumption of salt, sugar, saturated fat, and trans-fats which all act as preservatives together with chemical additives which increase the taste and consistency of the food. Processed food has a deficiency of fibre, essential fatty acids, vitamins, minerals, and phytochemicals. While the nutrients in processed food are decreased the shelf life and profits to the food industry are greatly increased.

The effect of the high animal and high processed food diet on health is an increased risk of all the non-communicable (non-infectious) diseases which are common in the USA but rare in Hunza. These include Cardiovascular disease (including, hypertension, heart attacks and strokes.) gallstones, kidney stones, peptic ulcer, hiatus hernia, appendicitis, colitis, constipation, haemorrhoids, varicose veins, fibroids, polycystic ovaries, endometriosis, infertility, miscarriage, birth defects, diabetes, thyroid problems, acne, osteoarthritis, osteoporosis, gout, mental health problems, dementia, auto-immune disease, allergies and cancer of every type.

Another nutritional pioneer who reinforces McCarrison's message was Denis Burkitt. Denis Burkitt, like McCarrison qualified as a doctor in Dublin but about 30 years later. He started work as a surgeon and General Practitioner in Uganda in 1946. He observed that the Africans had a markedly reduced incidence of bowel problems, obesity, diabetes, coronary heart disease and cancer compared with the UK and USA. He noted that the Africans produced greater quantity and softer faeces than people in the West and the absence of constipation was due to their consumption of much larger quantities of fibre rich vegetables. He hypothesised that a major cause of western disease was the consumption of refined carbohydrates with its low content of fibre.

In 1966 Burkitt left Uganda to take up a position at the Medical Research Council in London. He launched a worldwide crusade to increase our consumption of vegetable fibre. I had the privilege of attending one of his lectures in the 1970's. He gave an excellent talk with many informative slides. His quotations are very wise and memorable, so I have added a few.

"In Africa, treating people who live largely off the land on vegetables they grow, I hardly ever saw cases of many of the most common diseases in the United States and England- including coronary heart disease, adult-onset diabetes, varicose veins, obesity, diverticulitis, appendicitis, gallstones, dental cavities, haemorrhoids, hiatal hernias, and constipation. Western diets are so low on bulk and so dense in calories, that our intestines just don't pass enough volume to remain healthy."

"Diseases can rarely be eliminated through early diagnosis or good treatment, but prevention can eliminate disease."

"The only way we are going to reduce disease, is to go backward to the diets and lifestyles of our ancestors."

"The frying pan you should give to your enemy. Food should not be prepared in fat. Our bodies are adapted to a stone age diet of roots and vegetables."

"America is a constipated nation ... if you pass small stools, you have to have large hospitals."

"Western doctors are like poor plumbers. They treat a splashing tube by cleaning up the water. These plumbers are extremely apt at drying up the water, constantly inventing new, expensive and refined methods of drying up water. Somebody should teach them how to close the tap."

"If people are constantly falling off a cliff, you could place ambulances under the cliff or build a fence on top of the cliff. We are placing all too many ambulances under the cliff."

All quotations by Denis Burkitt MD, FRCS, FRS (1911 – 1993)

18

Analysis of Hunza and US diet

In the 1920's there were no recorded cases of heart attacks, diabetes, or cancer in Hunza. Most people lived a long life and were healthy in old age rather than suffering from the many western illnesses that were brought on by a poor diet. At that time the Hunza diet consisted of 1% animal products while the USA diet consisted of 48% animal products.

Complex carbohydrates mainly from vegetables made up 73% of the Hunza diet but only about 40% of the USA diet. Refined sugar made the total carbohydrate consumption 50% in the USA. Protein made up 10% of the Hunza diet and was mainly from plants while protein made up 15% of the USA diet and was mainly from animals.

Fat made up about 17% of the Hunza diet and was mainly monounsaturated and polyunsaturated from plants. Fat made up about 35% of the USA diet and was mainly saturated fat from animals (meat and dairy).

The animal products, especially butter, cheese and eggs contained high levels of cholesterol.

The Hunza diet is plant based with very small amounts of meat, butter, and cheese but no eggs. There is no cholesterol in plants. The monounsaturated and polyunsaturated fat in plants lower cholesterol levels and certain phytochemicals called phytosterols in plants also lower cholesterol levels.

The main difference is that the USA diet has a far greater proportion of animal products and processed food.

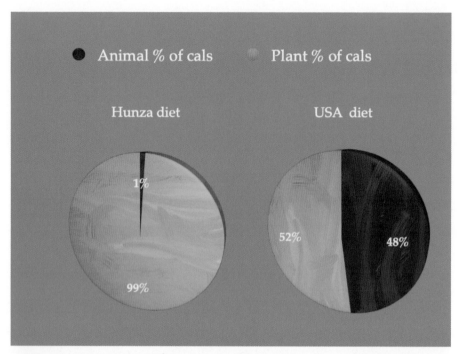

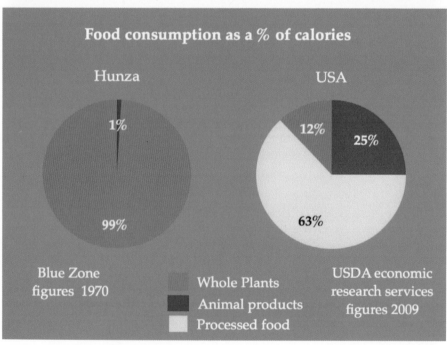

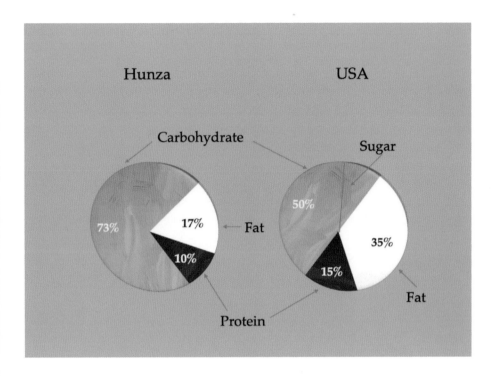

19

The Blue Zones

Hunza is one of the Blue Zones which are areas in the world where the people are exceptionally healthy and live long lives. They were chosen after research in the 1970's by Dr Alexander Leaf, a professor of clinical medicine at Harvard University in the USA. He was commissioned by the National Geographic

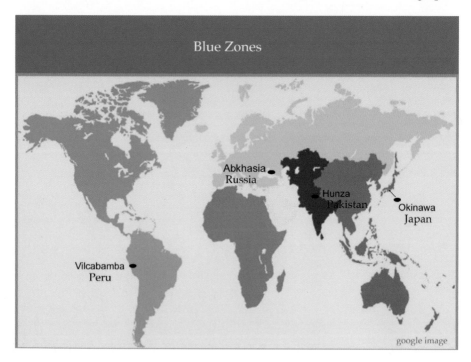

magazine to share with the world his observations and comparisons of those areas of the planet which were famous for longevity and health of their inhabitants. After many travels he choose four areas. Hunza then in Pakistan, Vilcabamba in Peru, Abkhazia in Russia and Okinawa in Japan.

In all these areas the incidence of cardiovascular disease, diabetes and cancer were extremely low and obesity rare. As well as a low incidence of physical illness there was an extremely low incidence of mental health problems, addiction, and crime. All these Blue Zone areas had a high carbohydrate, plant-based diet with over 80% of their diet from plants. Less than 20% of their diet was from animals. In Okinawa the main animal food eaten was freshly cooked fish. At the same time the incidence of all physical and mental problems was high in the USA. Only 48% of their diet was from plants and 52% was from animals. They also had a lot more refined carbohydrate and processed food.

	Abkhasia	Vilcabamba	Hunza	Okinawa	USA
CVD	Low	Low	Low	Low	High
Diabetes	Low	Low	Low	Low	High
Cancer	Low	Low	Low	Low	High
Obesity	Low	Low	Low	Low	High
Psychiatric	Low	Low	Low	Low	High
Addiction	Low	Low	Low	Low	High
Crime	Low	Low	Low	Low	High
% of diet Plants	90%	99%	99%	84%	48%
% of diet Animals	10%	1%	1%	16%	52%
Salt intake	Low	Low	Low	Low	High
Sugar intake	0	0	0	Low	High
Processed food	0	0	0	Low	High

CVD = Cardiovascular disease

20

Modern advances in nutrition

McCarrison would have known very little about some important discoveries concerning nutrition since his time.

a) The Methylation cycle: This is very complex but shows that certain nutrients are required for methylation which is required to synthesise new DNA and neurotransmitters.

b) Phytochemical's: (or phytonutrients) which have only been known about since the 1950's.

c) Prostaglandins: were first discovered in 1935 but very little was known about them until the 1980's when it was established that they were made from the essential fatty acid's omega 6 and omega 3.

d) Genetics: Geneticists have found the human genome to be far more complex than they at first thought and epigenetics' has shown that environmental factors such as diet can switch off or on the effect of many genes.

e) The Gut microbiome: Scientists have established that the enormous number of harmless bacteria in our gut have an important place in converting food to chemicals which help the immune system and help to synthesise neurotransmitters such as serotonin.

These new discoveries did not detract from McCarrison's observations and conclusions on diet but only served to support his case.

(a) The Methylation cycle

Methylation is required to make new neurotransmitters and DNA in the body daily. The amino acid Methionine is required for methylation. Methionine is an essential amino acid which cannot be synthesised by the body and must be obtained from the diet. It is present in larger amounts in animal than plant protein. In the process of methylation, the 'Meth' portion is removed which eventually results in the formation of homocysteine.

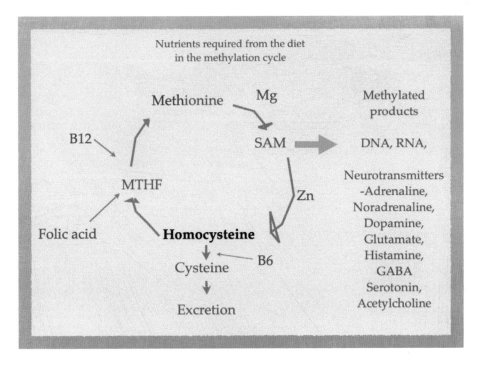

The homocysteine is then recycled to methionine but requires adequate Vitamin B12 and Folic acid to do this. Neurotransmitters are chemicals that enable communication between nerve cells in the brain and nervous system. They are created from various amino acids in animal and plant protein. They then require methylation to make them active.

An adequate supply of methionine from the diet is important to provide sufficient neurotransmitters and DNA. However, an excess of methionine together with any delay in the methylation cycle will cause an increase in homocysteine levels. A high homocysteine level (above 12 mmol/l) degrades elastin and collagen in arteries which increases the risk of cardiovascular disease such as heart attacks, strokes, and dementia. The degrading of collagen in bones increases the risk of osteoporosis, fractures, and osteoarthritis. Inadequate methylation of neurotransmitters increases the risk of mental health problems such as depression, attention deficit and hyperactivity disorder, schizophrenia, and bi-polar disorder. Addiction to stimulants of neurotransmitters such as caffeine, nicotine, cocaine, heroin, and amphetamines is made more likely if there is a deficiency of the nutrients that make or methylate neurotransmitters.

Inadequate methylation of DNA increases the risk of miscarriage, birth defects and cancer.

Animal protein has much higher levels of methionine than plant protein. Highest methionine levels are in eggs, then cheese and dairy products.

Beans including the Soya bean are the best sources of methionine in plants. Meat and fish have higher levels than beans, seeds, and nuts.

Cow's milk has twice as much methionine as soy milk.

Chicken has about 12 times as much as tofu (soya). Parmesan cheese has about 13 times as much as tofu.

Delay in the methylation cycle may be due to genetic deficiency of certain enzymes but is more commonly due to lack of certain nutrients from the diet. There is no vitamin B12 in plants and very little folic acid in animal products. People who eat a high animal protein, low plant carbohydrate diet may have an excess of methionine, plenty of B12 and zinc but a deficiency of folic acid and magnesium. People on a high plant based, low animal protein diet may have plenty of folic acid but a deficiency of methionine, B12 and zinc. In the early history of humans, the ability to make a fire and cook a small amount of meat and fish must have caused an increase in methionine, B12 and essential fatty acids. This would help to methylate neurotransmitters and possibly led to brain development and increased intelligence.

For the methylation cycle to work well it is important to have sufficient folic acid. Folic acid is a water-soluble B vitamin which is excreted within a few hours and the body stores are limited. It is in green leafy vegetables, root

Food	Methionine (mg/100g)
Animal	
Cheese (parmesan)	971
Cheese (cheddar)	661
Salmon	631
Lean Beef	572
Egg (one)	392
Plant	
Peanuts	289
Soybeans	224
Rice	167
Potato	33
Tomato	8
Apple	2

vegetables, mushrooms, beans, nuts and fruit. There is very little in meat, fish, eggs, dairy or processed food. Overcooking can reduce the amount of folic acid in food. Five servings of fruit or vegetables are required to guarantee the recommended dose of 400 micrograms daily. It is estimated that most people in western countries are deficient in folic acid especially old people and people with mental health problems. In one study 80% of old people admitted to hospital were deficient in folic acid.

In 1970 Dr Richard Smithells a paediatrician in the UK reported a link between insufficient folic acid and the occurrence of Spina Bifida in newborn babies. It took 20 years before his work was taken seriously. In 1992 the US and UK governments for the first time recommended a nutritional supplement. Pregnant women were advised to take 400 micrograms of folic acid daily. However, many women do not realise they are pregnant for the very early weeks and this is the time that the baby's spine and nervous system are developing. Spina bifida is a defect in spinal development which leaves no protection over the spinal nerves and this can lead to many problems including

Food average portions	B12 micrograms	Folate micrograms	B6 mg
Animal			
Chicken breast	trace	7	0.55
Sirloin steak (8oz)	5	35	1.08
Beefburger	1	4	0.11
Lambs liver fried	33	104	0.21
Cheddar cheese	0.4	13	0.04
Egg boiled	0.6	20	0.06
Plant			
Broccoli	nil	29	0.05
Potatoes boiled	nil	46	0.58
White bread 2 slices	nil	12	0.06
Wholemeal bread (2)	nil	30	0.1
Baked beans	nil	30	0.19
Peanuts	nil	30	0.31
Recommended daily	**1 to 6**	**200 to 400**	**2**

poor mobility and bladder control. The US government wisely added folic acid to refined white flour by law in 1998 and folic acid supplements to refined bread have now been introduced in over 70 countries including at last the UK in 2021.

Folic acid supplements in early pregnancy have reduced occurrences of Spina Bifida by about 70 %. They have also reduced the risk of all birth defects, congenital abnormalities, miscarriages and premature births. Apart from the benefits in pregnancy, folic acid supplements have been found to reduce the risk of cardiovascular disease, mental health disorders, anaemia, infertility and cancer.

(b) Phytochemical's

Phytochemicals are now recognised as a vital component of our diet. In total over 25,000 phytochemicals' have been discovered, and in most cases, they are concentrated in the colourful parts of plants like fruits, vegetables, nuts, legumes and wholegrains. Phytochemicals can also be called phytonutrients or polyphenols. Their role in plants is to protect them from insects, fungi, parasites and the sun. The red plants like tomatoes contain lycopene. Other red plants contain quercetin, hesperidin and anthocyanidins or may have a number of these phytochemicals. Blue plants may contain resveratrol, anthocyanidins, phenolics and flavonoids. Green plants may contain lutein, zeaxanthin, isoflavones, isothiocynates and sulphoraphane. White plants may contain allicin, quercetin, insoles and glucosinolates. Orange plants may contain alpha and beta-carotene, beta-cryptoxanthin, lutein, zeaxanthin and hesperidin. These phytochemicals are powerful antioxidants and are important for the health of all parts of the body including arteries, eyes, bones and brain. They are particularly important in supporting the immune system which reduces the risk of serious infection, auto-immune disease and cancer. Some phytochemicals are similar to cholesterol (phytosterols) but reduce blood levels of cholesterol as they compete with the harmful cholesterol from animals. This reduces the risk of cardiovascular disease. In a similar way another phytochemical called phytoestrogen in plants is like oestrogen but much weaker. By competing with the much stronger oestrogen in dairy products it reduces oestrogen blood levels. This reduces the risk of breast cancer.

In the 1920's at the time of Robert McCarrison's stay in Hunza there were no reported cases of cancer and I suspect that the amount and variety of phytochemical's consumed had a great deal to do with this fact.

An American businessman saw an opportunity to exploit and profit from the fact that cancer was becoming common in the USA but was rare in Hunza. His adverts pronounced that "The people of Hunza valley are the only people in the world without cancer because they use and eat apricot seeds, which contain vitamin B17, that kill cancer cells and strengthen the immune system." Amygdalin was thought to be the active anti-cancer compound isolated from the seeds of apricots. It was falsely claimed to be a vitamin but could more correctly be classified as a phytochemical.

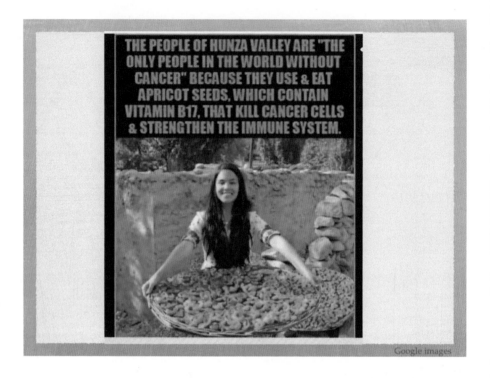

THE PEOPLE OF HUNZA VALLEY ARE "THE ONLY PEOPLE IN THE WORLD WITHOUT CANCER" BECAUSE THEY USE & EAT APRICOT SEEDS, WHICH CONTAIN VITAMIN B17, THAT KILL CANCER CELLS & STRENGTHEN THE IMMUNE SYSTEM.

Google images

In 1961 Laetrile a semisynthetic derivative of amygdalin was patented and heavily promoted as an anti-cancer drug. It sold well despite side effects from the fact that metabolism turned the product into cyanide and poisoned some patients. It was not until 1977 that controlled, blinded trials suggested that it had no more anti-cancer activity than placebo. The promotion of Laetrile to treat cancer has been described in the medical literature as an example of quackery and as "the slickest, most sophisticated, and certainly the most re-munerative cancer quack promotion in medical history."

There is still a tendency for the pharmaceutical industry to search for an individual phytochemical with anti-cancer properties and then patent it. I suspect that the truth is, that many of the thousands of phytochemicals have anti-cancer properties, but they probably work in a synergistic way and may not be as effective if isolated.

The effort to find anticancer agents from plants was launched by the US National Cancer Institute (NCI) in 1957. Since then, more than 35.000 plant species have been investigated. This has resulted in the discovery of many

anticancer drugs such as vincristine, vinblastine, and taxol. It has been estimated that the plant kingdom comprises of approximately 250,000 species
and only about 10% have been studied for the treatment of various diseases. It
is estimated that about 60% of clinically approved anticancer drugs are deriva-
tives of herbal plants which have been used as treatment for many ailments
over many hundreds of years.

(c) Prostaglandins

Prostaglandins are Chemical messengers which are synthesized in almost every cell of the body and act within that cell. They are not stored and have a short effect before they are metabolized and excreted. They are created from the essential fatty acids omega 6 and omega 3 which cannot be synthesized by the body so have to be provided in the diet. Omega-6 is mainly from seeds and nuts and animals if fed on grain. They produce a mixture of inflammatory and anti-inflammatory prostaglandins. The inflammatory prostaglandins come mainly from animal products and have harmful effects unless they are balanced by sufficient Omega-3 which is purely anti-inflammatory.

If the diet is top heavy in inflammatory prostaglandins it causes the arteries to constrict raising blood pressure, and the airways to constrict causing asthma. It increases the risk of blood clotting. In the stomach it increases acid and decreases the protective mucous. It can cause the bowel and uterus to contract. It decreases kidney function. It increases eye pressure, suppresses

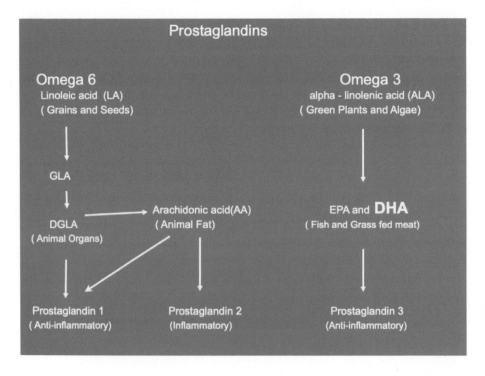

the immune system, and increases pain and inflammation. Anti-inflammatory prostaglandins have the opposite effect.

Many prostaglandins have been identified and synthesized for use in several medical problems. This gives an indication of how powerful their effects can be. Synthetic prostaglandins are used to lower eye pressure in glaucoma (e.g. latanoprost, travoprost, bimatoprost), to dilate blood vessels in newborns with congenital heart disease and treat erectile dysfunction in men (e.g. alprostadil), to prevent stomach ulcers in patients taking non-steroidal anti-inflammatory drugs such as aspirin and ibuprofen (e.g. misoprostol), to soften the cervix for induction of labour (e.g. dinoprostone) and to induce an abortion in the early stages of pregnancy (E2).

Small amounts of essential fats (omega 3 and omega 6) are present in grains, fresh green plants and nuts but are removed when foods are processed. The reason that wholegrain bread becomes stale much faster than white bread is largely down to the removal of omega-3 from white bread to give it greater shelf life. By far the best source of omega-3 is from fish but it is also present in

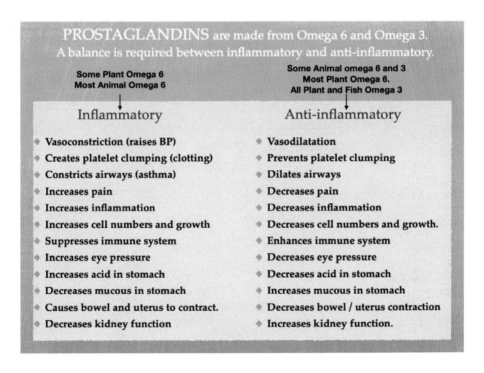

PROSTAGLANDINS are made from Omega 6 and Omega 3.
A balance is required between inflammatory and anti-inflammatory.

Some Plant Omega 6 Most Animal Omega 6	Some Animal omega 6 and 3 Most Plant Omega 6. All Plant and Fish Omega 3
Inflammatory	Anti-inflammatory
◆ Vasoconstriction (raises BP)	◆ Vasodilatation
◆ Creates platelet clumping (clotting)	◆ Prevents platelet clumping
◆ Constricts airways (asthma)	◆ Dilates airways
◆ Increases pain	◆ Decreases pain
◆ Increases inflammation	◆ Decreases inflammation
◆ Increases cell numbers and growth	◆ Decreases cell numbers and growth.
◆ Suppresses immune system	◆ Enhances immune system
◆ Increases eye pressure	◆ Decreases eye pressure
◆ Increases acid in stomach	◆ Decreases acid in stomach
◆ Decreases mucous in stomach	◆ Increases mucous in stomach
◆ Causes bowel and uterus to contract.	◆ Decreases bowel / uterus contraction
◆ Decreases kidney function	◆ Increases kidney function.

grass fed meat. In Hunza, people very rarely ate fish, but they obtained a good balance of essential fats because of the large amount of wholegrain bread and fresh vegetables they ate, and any meat was grass fed. In the USA they often have an excess of grain fed meat and processed food which are high in omega 6 but deficient in Omega 3. A diet high in inflammatory prostaglandins increases the risk of hypertension, heart attacks, strokes, glaucoma, peptic ulcer, asthma, irritable bowel, painful periods, miscarriage, reduced kidney function, infection and cancer. The correct balance of essential fats is also important for good mental health and an inflammatory diet may cause learning difficulties, depression, aggression and other mental health problems, which increase the risk of addiction and crime.

(d) Genetics

DNA (Deoxyribonucleic Acid) is a molecule that contains the hereditary information for making new cells. Chromosomes are thread like structures consisting of protein and a single molecule of DNA. They are present in the nucleus of all animal and plant cells. Each cell in the human body has twenty-three pairs of chromosomes. A total of forty-six.

Half of these come from the mother and half from the father. Two of the chromosomes X and Y determine whether you are male or female at birth. Females have two copies of the X chromosome (XX) and males have one X and one Y (XY). In 1953 James Watson and Francis Crick discovered the structure of DNA. The twisted ladder structure was named the double helix. It opened the way for research into understanding how genes control the chemical processes in the human body. Genes are segments of DNA that contain the instructions for making a specific protein. Each chromosome contains thousands of genes. Each of the estimated 30,000 genes in the human genome makes an average of three proteins. In 2003 the Human Genome Project was completed after about 20 years of effort. This was an international research effort to determine the DNA sequence of the entire human genome. This has led to a much better understanding of how genes control the body metabolism but there is still a great deal that we do not understand. One of the complicating factors was the discovery of epigenetics. This was a hypothesis in the 1940's but was not defined until the 1990's. Epigenetics is the change in gene activity or expression that can occur without any structural change in the underlying DNA or genes. Environmental factors such as diet and methylation can make certain genes behave differently. These epigenetic changes can become permanent in a human and inherited by their children. However, the changes can be reversed. It was hoped that we would be able to predict human disorders by understanding the role of each gene, but epigenetics' makes this much more complicated. Some medical problems such as Huntingdon's disease or Cystic Fibrosis are due to inheriting a defective gene but the common western illnesses such as cardiovascular disease, adult-onset diabetes and cancer are rarely linked to a particular gene. Only about 5% of cancers are linked to a faulty inherited gene. The most well-known genes are the BRCA (BReast

CAncer) genes. Most people do not realise that everyone has these genes, and they play an important part in suppressing cell mutation and tumour formation. It is only if people inherit or develop a faulty gene that the risk of certain cancers is increased. These genes are more likely to become faulty if DNA methylation is upset or the immune system is inadequate.

(e) The Gut Microbiome

It is estimated that there are about 1,000 different species of bacteria in the human's large bowel and a total of about 40 trillion bacteria. Together with viruses and fungi they make up the gut microbiome. Recent research has shown that the gut microbiome plays an important part in keeping us healthy. It breaks down food with its digestive enzymes and provides protection from harmful bacteria and toxins in food. It produces short chain fatty acids from the fermentation of indigestible fibre. These fatty acids stimulate immune cell activity which reduces the risk of colon cancer. They also help with regulating blood sugar and cholesterol levels. They influence appetite and help bile break down fat. The bacteria also help with the creation of certain vitamins, amino acids and neurotransmitters such as serotonin. The health of the gut biome is improved by having a mainly plant based diet of fruits, vegetables, beans, nuts and whole grains with plenty of nutrients and fibre. Animal based diets such as meat have less important nutrients, often contain antibiotics and have no fibre.

21

Cancer: possible causes and treatment

For many years chemotherapy and radiotherapy have been the main treatments for cancer. They both destroy rapidly dividing cells such as cancer cells but both may also damage normal cells and can cause severe side effects. Immunotherapy is becoming more popular either on its own or together with the other therapies as it is often more effective and usually has less severe side effects.. Immunotherapy drugs help the immune system to destroy cancer cells in a more natural way. They include phytochemical's and man-made monoclonal antibodies which were introduced in the 1980's. The monoclonal antibodies have a very similar effect to phytochemicals on the immune system. They both help to remove cells with damaged DNA and reduce cancer cell growth. Both have an effect in blocking the growth of new blood vessels (angiogenesis). The monoclonal antibodies are often more powerful but much more expensive and have far more side effects.

"For every drug that benefits a patient, there is a natural substance that can achieve the same effect." Quote by Carl Pfeiffer – American pharmacologist (1908 – 1988)

The cells in our body are constantly dying and being renewed. The DNA which forms each new cell can be damaged by toxins and poor nutrition which may lead to mutant cancer cells being formed. Cancer was rare in Hunza in the early 1900's not because of genetics but because there were very

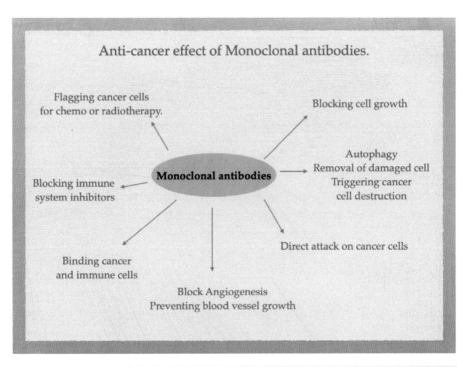

Anti-cancer effect of Monoclonal antibodies.

Flagging cancer cells for chemo or radiotherapy.

Blocking cell growth

Monoclonal antibodies

Autophagy
Removal of damaged cell
Triggering cancer
cell destruction

Blocking immune system inhibitors

Binding cancer and immune cells

Direct attack on cancer cells

Block Angiogenesis
Preventing blood vessel growth

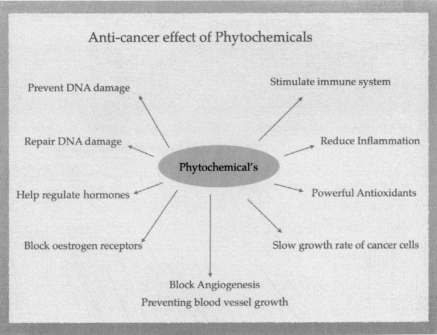

Anti-cancer effect of Phytochemicals

Prevent DNA damage

Stimulate immune system

Repair DNA damage

Reduce Inflammation

Phytochemical's

Help regulate hormones

Powerful Antioxidants

Block oestrogen receptors

Slow growth rate of cancer cells

Block Angiogenesis
Preventing blood vessel growth

few environmental toxins and they had an excellent diet which formed healthy DNA and provided a very strong immune system which removed any abnormal cells. It is thought that humans as they get older often develop small clumps of cancer cells. These start off about the size of a grain of sand and unless they can develop a blood supply and grow, they cause no harm. Angiogenic factors produce sprouting capillaries from the nearest artery. This supplies the clump of cancer cells with oxygen and nutrients and enables it to grow into a larger tumour and eventually metastasise. The main angiogenic factors are thought to be Insulin growth factor (IGF), human growth factor (HGF), Insulin and inflammatory prostaglandins. Insulin Growth Factor, Human Growth Factor and inflammatory prostaglandins are present in much larger amounts in animal products such as meat and dairy while refined sugar in processed food produces much higher insulin levels than natural carbohydrate sugars. The USA diet therefore has far more products that promote angiogenesis while the Hunza diet has far more anti-angiogenic phytochemicals. Scientists, Colin Campbell in his book 'The China Study' and Jane Plant in her book 'Your life in your hands' strongly support the view that an excess of animal protein and hormones from meat and especially dairy products are largely responsible for the increase in cancer in the USA and Western countries. Thomas Colin Campbell was Professor Emeritus of Nutritional Biochemistry at Cornell University USA. In his excellent book 'The China Study' he reported on his research into cancer of the liver in Filipino children. It was thought that the high consumption of aflatoxin, a fungal mould toxin found in peanuts and corn caused the problem. Aflatoxin is one of the most potent carcinogens ever discovered. It was thought that reducing malnutrition in the poor by giving them more protein would decrease the risk of liver cancer but instead they found that children with the highest protein intake had the greatest risk of cancer. Animal studies indicated that low protein diets inhibited the initiation of cancer by aflatoxin, regardless of how much of this carcinogen was administered. The proteins that promoted cancer were animal proteins especially casein the protein in milk. Plant proteins did not promote cancer. Jane Plant was a Professor of Geochemistry at Imperial college London. She developed breast cancer at a young age and noted the low incidence of breast cancer in Chinese women compared with those in the UK and USA. Chinese women in the 1960's had a very low consumption of milk and dairy products. The dairy industry had not developed in China at that time and the people were thought to be mainly lactose intolerant. She discovered a correlation between cancer rate and dairy consumption. She commented "basically dairy has now got a lot of oestrogen in it because it's common practice to milk pregnant cows, which has driven up the oestrogen content of milk. It also contains tiny proteins called growth factors, and these growth factors directly promote cancer." She recommended that cancer patients take conventional treatment but also adopt a dairy free diet. Although her ideas were not accepted by the medical establishment, many women benefited from taking her advice. I would like to make it clear that I am not advocating that better nutrition is a substitute for conventional cancer treatments which are often very successful. Nutrition's main role is in preventing disease, but it can also help to secure a more successful outcome when used together with conventional treatment. Nutrition should not be considered as an alternative treatment but as a complimentary treatment with a strong scientific basis. We will never be able to dispense with

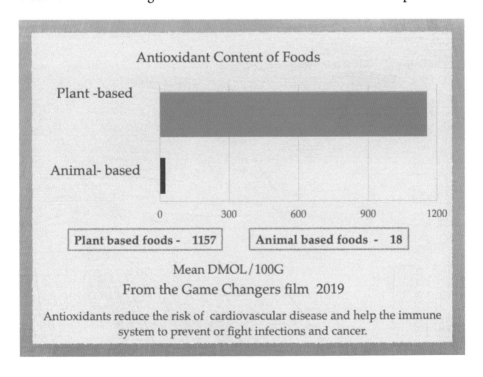

Antioxidant Content of Foods

Plant -based

Animal- based

0   300   600   900   1200

Plant based foods - 1157   Animal based foods - 18

Mean DMOL / 100G

From the Game Changers film 2019

Antioxidants reduce the risk of cardiovascular disease and help the immune system to prevent or fight infections and cancer.

all modern drugs and vaccines but with better nutrition there is the possibility of prevention and of reducing the amount of medication and other treatments in almost all illnesses.

As shown in the slide above, plant-based foods (especially fresh whole vegetables and fruit) have far more antioxidants than animal based foods and these antioxidants have a major effect in supporting the immune system and preventing cancer.

22

Thoughts on diets and supplements

The number of vegans is increasing but it is difficult for them to get enough vitamin B12 and essential fatty acids such as omega-3 from natural products so they are advised to take supplements. Vitamin B12 is plentiful in animal products and only required in small amounts as unlike other B vitamins it can be stored in the liver. There is no B12 in plants. The best source of omega-3 is from fish. I think that any diet that requires supplements is not an ideal diet. A lot of people in the USA realise that they have a poor diet and so over half of the population take multivitamins, multi minerals or other supplements. Some of these supplements do more harm than good as it is easy to take an excess of certain ingredients. The people in Hunza never needed any supplements and they would not have been available anyway until the late 1930's when vitamins were first synthesised. Nature is much better at providing the correct mixture of nutrients than any chemist. The mixture of protein, carbohydrate, fat, vitamins, minerals and phytochemicals is extremely complex, and we still have a lot to learn about how they interact. The Hunza diet in the 1920s produced people with excellent mental as well as physical health. They were noted for their calm and pleasant mood but exactly how this occurred is complicated. The Hunza people had an excellent mainly plant based diet which was rich in vitamins, minerals, essential fatty acids and phytochemicals, many of which are essential for good brain function and protective against mental illness but there may have been additional nutritional factors that we know very little about. For example, mineral laden silt produced by the glaciers could provide more lithium in the soil and therefore plants than is usual. This is the same lithium that is used in batteries. It is also used to treat the mania of bipolar disorder as it has a mood calming effect. It is normal to find it in all soils, but the amount varies. A recent scientific paper gave the interesting information that there is a great deal more lithium in plant foods than animal foods. The mean lithium content (micrograms per gram dry weight) of foodstuffs was given as follows:

Plants foods – Nuts 8.8, Cereals 4.4, Vegetables 2.3.
Animal foods – Fish 3.1, Dairy 0.5, Meat 0.012.

The refining of processed food would remove most minerals including lithium.

The overriding message is that humans should eat whole foods and mainly plants. A small amount of meat and fish to supply adequate B12 and Omega 3 is sensible. For example, a grilled lean fillet steak and a portion of fresh fish could be afforded if both were eaten once a week instead of having a fried beefburger, chicken or bacon every day. A small amount of dairy products such as milk, butter, cheese and yogurt can be consumed without harm but an excess provides too much cholesterol, saturated fat, growth and sex hormones.

At present cheap subsidised cheese is often added to almost every fast food. The mixture of fat from cheese and refined carbohydrate from a white bread roll as in a burger, or cheese and white pasta flour as in a pizza, is very tasty especially with added salt (food chemists would say it has "the bliss factor"). Because the white bread is refined, sugar gets absorbed quickly and insulin levels rise to keep the blood sugar levels down, The fat in cheese causes resistance to the effect of insulin, so that even more insulin has to be produced. This increases the risk of developing diabetes. Eggs are nutritious but have a lot of cholesterol and it is not advisable to have them too often.

In my opinion all foods can contribute to a healthy diet if they are not consumed in too large a quantity or to frequently. The human body is amazing at coping with unhealthy food and small amounts of toxins. Processed food in small amounts can be acceptable if balanced by an otherwise healthy diet.

Examples of processed foods include white bread, cola drinks, sweets, milk chocolate, ice-cream, crisps, cakes, and biscuits. Most processed foods provide tasty calories but very little nutrition. The body strives for the missing nutrients by increasing the appetite and this may cause obesity.

In a recent experiment by the National Institute for Health USA (2019) twenty healthy young adults agreed to live in a clinic setting for 28 days so their food intake could be closely monitored. For 14 days, subjects received either an ultra-processed diet or a minimally processed diet, then they were switched to the other diet for 14 days. In both cases they were allowed to eat as much or as little as they wanted. Subjects on the ultra-processed diet consumed 500 calories more per day and gained two pounds more in weight. When switched to the minimally processed diet for 14 days they consumed 500 less calories a day and lost two pounds in weight. This largely explains the high incidence of obesity in Western countries.

A low carbohydrate, high protein diet such as the Keto or Atkins type diet slips in and out of popularity for losing weight. In the short term it seems to work well especially for obese diabetics. Less carbohydrate and therefore sugar is consumed and so naturally less insulin is required and blood sugar levels go down. The fluid associated with the storage of glycogen is lost and the patient feels elated by the 'methionine rush' from the high animal protein and weight loss. The lack of glucose in the diet means the glycogen stores become empty and so fat is metabolised to produce ketones for energy instead of glucose. The brain and muscles can use ketones for energy, but they prefer glucose as it is more effective. Athletes preparing for a marathon consume a large amount of carbohydrate before a race to build up their glycogen stores so that plenty of glucose is available to give the most efficient energy supply for the brain as well as muscles. Long term the low carbohydrate-high protein diet is bad for your health as it increases the risk of almost all the common western illnesses. The lack of fibre causes constipation and reduced immunity. The high animal fat and cholesterol content increases the risk of cardiovascular disease and gallstones. The high animal protein content increases the risk of kidney stones, osteoporosis, osteoarthritis, and many other problems. If people need to lose weight they just need to eat less of a healthy whole food, plant-based diet.

23

Food efficiency, resources and climate change

Reducing our consumption of animal products would not only improve our personal health but improve the health of the Earth.

It is estimated that a meat-based diet requires 18 times more land than a vegan diet. Deforestation occurs mainly to provide crops such as soya which are used to feed animals rather than humans.

As well as consuming a great deal of food animals drink a great deal of water. It is estimated that it takes less water to produce a year's food for a vegan than to produce a month's food for a meat-eater.

Billions of land animals are killed for food each year and in the search for profit many are treated badly. These animals consume most of the rich nations grain and water which would be better used by humans in poor countries. They produce a great deal of waste especially if confined to barns and large animals in particular produce methane which is a major source of greenhouse gas emissions and climate change. The message is starting to be heard through better education and increased knowledge and I hope this trend continues.

24

Conclusion

In this book I have used Hunza in the 1920's as an example of a poor country with no scientific knowledge of nutrition but a diet which has evolved over many hundreds of years and has proven to be healthy.

In comparison to Hunza there was much greater scientific knowledge of nutrition in rich countries such as the USA in the 1920's. Unfortunately, this knowledge was often ignored or suppressed as it conflicted with the profits of very powerful industries. These include the meat, dairy, sugar, and processed food industries. The advertising industry became very clever at marketing the products of these industries and the medical and pharmaceutical industries have profited from the poor health of the population. To its credit the USA allows critics to voice their opinions and I have obtained a lot of my information from US authors and data. Many people have improved their diets because of this information, but most people are still not well informed or confused.

I realise that the situation today in Hunza will be different as they now have a thriving tourist industry and have become wealthier and better educated. I have no doubt that the people will inevitably have been influenced by western values and diet.

The only way that the situation can change in the Western countries is by providing more nutritional information to the public so they can choose a healthy diet. Education on nutrition should increase and improve for children, teachers, parents, chefs, doctors and nurses. Free healthy school meals for all school children would be worthwhile. Subsidies should be reduced on animal products and given for vegetables and fruit. Vending machines with cheap unhealthy snacks and drinks should be avoided in schools, workplaces and especially hospitals. Unhealthy snacks should not be placed near the checkout in shops. There should be a less stressful society with more people working shorter hours and with adequate pay.

A very poor diet can cause severe mental illness but more common is the suboptimal diet which causes a suboptimal mental state. This increases the risk of mild depression, anxiety, paranoia, delusions, addiction, and aggressive behaviour. If we could persuade more people to have a healthy diet, I am sure there would be less physical and mental illness. There would be less time taken off work and less early retirement on medical grounds. There would be less domestic abuse and divorces. There would be less addiction and crime. We would need less hospitals and prisons, less doctors, pharmacists, police, and lawyers. Above all it would reduce the suffering of those who develop physical and mental illnesses. Some industries would suffer reduced profits but having made so much profit in the past they could diversify. Overall, a healthier population is bound to improve a countries economy.

It was only after many years and only after overwhelming evidence that some doctors managed to convince politicians and the public that tobacco smoking could cause cancer and should take measures to reduce its consumption. Eventually despite intense lobbying from the tobacco industry it was reluctantly agreed by the politicians that people's health had greater priority than the profits of the tobacco industry and the resulting share of profits to the Inland revenue and shareholders.

Then as now, the public and politicians are reluctant to accept very convincing scientific evidence. The public is not keen to change a diet which it enjoys, and the politicians are under great pressure from profitable industries that pay a lot of tax. Even some doctors are not convinced that diet is a major factor in health which I find hard to believe. A recent online survey of 1005 American physicians by Medscape in August 2022 found that only 55% of them thought that their patients would benefit from advice on nutrition.

It may be that only if the public demand for healthy food increases that businesspeople and politicians will respond. I hope this book helps in that respect.

25

Bibliography

I qualified as a medical doctor in 1966 with a great deal of knowledge about how to diagnose and treat many diseases but very little knowledge of nutrition or how to prevent diseases.

Working as a GP in the 1970's I was given a book on nutrition by a patient.

It was a small book of about 100 pages called Health Hazards of a Western diet by Dr George A. Stanton. This book and a family history of coronary heart disease sparked my interest in nutrition and health.

Unfortunately, I was too busy dealing with the many western ailments to do any research of my own, but I have taken a strong interest ever since.

I have read far too many books on nutrition and give credit to the many nutritional pioneers who I have gained my knowledge from.

The many books include

'Health Hazards of a Western diet' by George A. Stanton
'Don't forget Fibre in your diet' by Denis Burkitt
'The Saccharine Disease. by T.L. Cleave
'Pure white and deadly' by John Yudkin
'Nutrition and Health' by Sir Robert McCarrison
'The Optimum Nutrition Bible' by Patrick Holford.
'Plant based nutrition and health' by Stephen Walsh

'Eating well for optimum health' by Andrew Weil

'Healthy at 100' by John Robbins

'The Food Revolution' by John Robbins

'The China Study' by T. Colin Campbell

'Whole' by T. Colin Campbell

'The Future of Nutrition' by T. Colin Campbell

'Prevent and Reverse Heart Disease' by Caldwell B.Esselstyn

'Reversing Heart Disease' by Dean Ornish

'50 ways to a healthy heart' by Prof. Christian Barnard

'Whitewash' by Joseph Keon

'Fast Food Nation' by Eric Schlosser.

'Your life in your hands' by Prof. Jane Plant

'Fat Chance; by Robert Lustig

'Catching Fire' by Richard Wranham

'Forks over Knives' by Gene Stone

'The Omnivore's Dilemma' by Michael Pollan

'How not to Die' by Michael Gregor

'Gut' by Giulia Enders

'The Diet Myth' by Tim Spector

'Spoon-Fed' by Tim Spector

'The Wheel of Health- The secret path of Hunza' by Guy T. Wrench and from many articles on the internet.

I have not included detailed references or an index as I do not think many readers use them and it would take another book to list them.

Printed in Great Britain
by Amazon

32357953R00057